Herbs that heal

HERBS THAT HEAL

William A. R. Thomson, M.D.

Illustrated by Yvonne Skargon

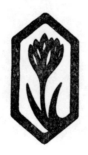

ADAM AND CHARLES BLACK · LONDON

First published 1976
A & C Black Limited
35 Bedford Row, London WC1R 4JH

© William A. R. Thomson, 1976

ISBN 0 7136 1688 1

Printed in Great Britain by
Hazell Watson & Viney Ltd,
Aylesbury, Bucks

Contents

Preface

> 'The apparently instinctive practice of taking drugs is believed to exist among the lower animals. It is a fascinating subject for the speculative mind to ponder how this instinct arose, and how, as primitive man struggled upwards, a belief in the power of drugs to remedy disease originated.'

So wrote Sir David Campbell in his inaugural lecture as Professor of Materia Medica in the University of Aberdeen in 1930. We are still speculating but there seems to be little doubt that as our ancestors issued forth through the mist of antiquity from prehistoric to historic times this belief was firmly ingrained in them, and today it is as strongly fixed as ever.

It is not the purpose of this book to discuss the philosophical implications of this belief, but rather to accept it and on that basis to delve into the problem of the current controversy between those who pin their faith to man-made drugs, and those who have more faith in the bounty of Nature. In many ways, like so many controversies it is a somewhat artificial one. What we require is a symbiosis between the synthesist and the naturalist – so admirably exemplified in the emblem designed by Mrs Vivienne Kenney for the British Pharmaceutical Conference in Nottingham in 1974, and reproduced on the title page. Essentially this is a purple crocus enclosed in a benzene ring to represent the association of the old herbal medicines with modern synthetic medicines.

What has happened in the last hundred years, however (with increasing crescendo during the past fifty years), is that, riding on the crest of the wave of scientific progress, the synthesists have taken the bit between their teeth and, with all the arrogance of scientists – than which there is none greater – have assumed that all new drugs must come from the laboratory.

Fortunately, their precipitate retiral to chromium-plated research institutes was slowed down by the introduction of penicillin from Nature and the need for the aid of Nature in the manufacture of cortisone and the sex hormones. The lesson, however, has only been fully appreciated by a minority of research workers, who realize that much more attention must be given to investigating the wealth of therapeutic possibilities that lie hidden in the secret fastnesses of Nature. The majority still hanker after the concept of tailoring drugs *de novo* to suit individual illnesses. The snag that is too often overlooked is that we do not know enough about the intricacies of the human body to be able to do this on a strictly scientific basis. There are too many imponderables and, as every scientist should realize, when dealing with so many unknowns science tends to be more misleading than helpful.

I am not certain that I am prepared to go as far as Goethe in his belief that 'nothing happens in living Nature that is not in relation to the whole', but I have a hunch that the integration of man with Nature as a whole is closer than many have suspected in the post-Darwinian era.

I am certainly no 'back-to-Nature' enthusiast, but the more I have delved into the history of drugs, the more convinced have I become that to ignore Nature is to ask for trouble. Again and again, as in the case of ergot in midwifery and of digitalis, the scientists have gone astray and, instead of improving upon Nature, have held up progress towards the better understanding of the working of valuable drugs.

What I have therefore done in this book is to try and present a balanced picture of what Nature has to supply in the way of herbs that heal. No attempt has been made to cover all the well-trodden ground. Thus, the stories of quinine and of opium are not included.

Much has had to be left out in order to keep the book to a reasonable size. Thus, herbs such as dandelion and horehound, which are asking for further investigation, have been omitted. Neither could I find space for the nettle, which always reminds me of my old friend, the blacksmith, at Farncombe in Surrey, whom I got to know well during the 1939–45 War. In his yard he had a magnificent clump of nettles, and I once asked him why he did not dig them up. He held out his old gnarled, rheumatic hands in reply. 'Doctor,' he said, 'when the rheumatics in my hands get too bad and I can't stand them any more, I plunge them into that bed of nettles, and the pain goes at once.' A drastic but effective, safe and cheap remedy.

My aim has been to pick out the more salient points, what might be described as the growing points, in an attempt to provide for the lay reader an over-all picture of the possibilities of progress, if only the synthesists and the naturalists will work hand in hand. As has been repeatedly shown, such collaboration can often improve upon Nature, provided the scientist is not too clever and does not carry purification too far. Here, as is not yet fully appreciated, there is an 'art' in the scientific study of drugs, just as much as there is a 'science' in the practice of medicine.

All in all, it has been a fascinating study. I have read widely, deliberately avoiding selection in order to get an over-all and, I trust, reasonably balanced picture. I have read some incredible statements, but herbalists are not unique in this respect. If only some of these claims were true, how much easier life would be for many of us. But I have always forgiven them as I became more and more immersed in all the wonders of Nature as revealed in the healing herbs with which she has supplied mankind from his earliest days. The list I have appended in the short bibliography at the end of the book is a highly selective one and merely meant as a guide to those who would like to probe more deeply into this world of herbs that heal.

It is a world that I leave reluctantly. I shall miss it, but console myself with the thought that 'there is rosemary, that's for remembrance', and hope that in the days to come she will not allow me to forget all that I have learned in my search for 'herbs that heal'.

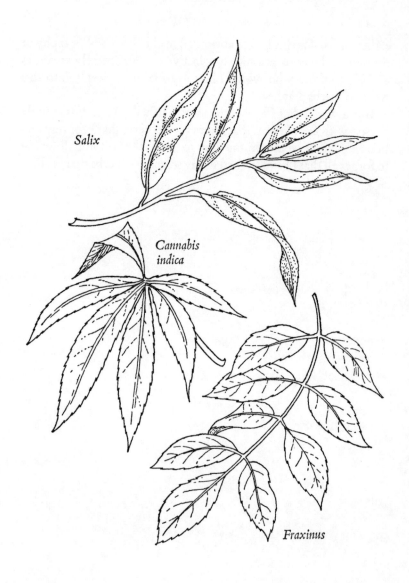

Salix

Cannabis
indica

Fraxinus

1

The herbal revolution

The quadrangle of the Medical School in the University of Edinburgh bears the superscription: *Ars longa vita brevis*. Alas, as in every medical school in the United Kingdom, and probably in the United States of America as well, the emphasis, so far as the curriculum is concerned, is all on the second part. In other words, medical students are trained, not educated. Nowhere in their curriculum is a place found for a consideration of the rhythms of life: night and day, sleeping and waking, summer and winter, seedtime and harvest, light and shade, sunshine and storm. The emphasis is all on the accumulation of facts and their short-term effects. Never is the student allowed, far less encouraged, to sit back and cogitate on the implications of life, where and how man fits into Nature, and to what extent this affects the quality as well as the quantity of life.

Never are they reminded of Wordsworth's outburst:

> 'The world is too much with us; late and soon,
> Getting and spending, we lay waste our powers:
> Little we see in Nature that is ours.'

Yet in Nature is to be found many a secret, the revealing of which has brought to light a healing drug, a soothing balm, or a solace to the distressed mind. Quinine, till well within living memory the only remedy for malaria; morphia, the pain-reliever *in excelsis* which the ingenuity of scientific man has failed to improve upon; emetine, still the most effective controller of amoebic dysentery; rauwolfia, which introduced the much abused concept of tranquillizers; curare, one of the most valuable handmaidens of modern anaesthesia, not to mention penicillin: all these we owe to Nature.

Many more could be added to the list, and are discussed later in this book. As Professor R E Schultz, the distinguished Harvard ethnobotanist has pointed out: 'Many are the instances where folk uses of plants, had they been seriously followed up, might have led much earlier to valuable discoveries'. Of two examples he mentions, one is 'the rediscovery of the use in Mexico and the exact botanical identification of several potent hallucinogens – especially the "sacred" mushrooms and morning glories – all fully outlined in detail in early historical chronicles and missionary reports'. The other is his comment that 'had we critically evaluated the writings of the Egyptian papyri, we might not have had to wait until the 1940s for an acquaintance with the antibiotic properties of certain fungi'.

Yet, with certain notable exceptions, all we did was to scoff at our forebears for their 'childish' faith in herbs, ridicule them for the fuss they made about collecting their herbs at a certain time of day, a certain season, or a certain period of the moon, and ended up by describing it all as an unholy, or holy, combination of magic, astrology and superstition. Typical of this attitude, though expressed in the statesman-like language of the holder of such a high office, are the views expressed by Sir Arnold Burgen, Director of the National Institute of Medical Research, London, in the Conference Lecture which he delivered to the British Pharmaceutical Conference in 1974. In the course of this, as reported in the *Pharmaceutical Journal*, he commented that the current 'back-to-Nature' movement was having an influence on society's attitude to drugs. That was evidenced by those people who said that all research should be stopped, that we knew all we needed to know and that we should go back to the primeval wisdom of folklore. But, surely, one did not wish to return to an era of ineffective drugs. In the future there could still be discoveries of further great life-saving drugs as there had been in the past with insulin, penicillin and the sulphonamides. The 'back-to-Nature' attitude supported tough legislation against the introduction of new drugs and was having a serious effect upon the attitude of pharmaceutical firms in looking for new compounds. In the USA practically all the drug companies had diversified into cosmetics, scientific apparatus, etc., because they were fearful that new legislation might seriously restrict new drug development.

But what do we find today? What kind of drugs are being produced by this 'fearful' pharmaceutical industry, and being prescribed by the present generation of doctors? According to Sir George Godber, the predecessor of the present Chief Medical Officer to the Department of Health and Social Security, in his 1975 Rock Carling Fellowship Lecture, 'the number of admissions to hospital for treatment of adverse reactions to drugs now exceeds 100,000 a year'. According to the *British Medical Journal*, side-effects have been reported in practically three-quarters of the patients receiving a drug widely prescribed for the treatment of high blood pressure, and there are no fewer than twenty different diuretics (stimulators of the secretion of urine) now available for prescription, the use of which by doctors in 1973 'suggested a substantial degree of inappropriate prescribing'. It added to this comment: 'Clearly a reminder of the real virtue of the simpler diuretics is timely'.

13

This danger of the current multiplicity of modern, synthetic, potent drugs is one that has been emphasized by Dr Halfden Mahler, the Danish Director-General of the World Health Organization. 'If you have to deal with 30,000 different types of drugs on the market in any particular country', he is reported as saying, 'it is quite impossible for any doctor to have sufficient knowledge.' In his opinion, 95% of illness could be cured by 100 to 200 drugs, a range with which the doctor could cope, but in most European countries he is confronted with 30,000 drugs or more.

Or again, there is the report from Glasgow which shows that among eighty-two deaths of patients seen at the University Centre for Rheumatic Diseases over a ten-year period, 'there was a disquieting number of deaths attributed to drug therapy'. But perhaps the most scathing commentary on current drug practice is that of Professor D G Webberley, of the Department of Pharmacy in the University of Aston:

'Can we be happy with a current advertisement, from a highly important drug company, showing a harassed mother scolding a child, which states: "Adverse circumstances such as too many children and too little money are recognized causes of neurotic depression or anxiety neurosis in persons with a low resistance to stress. These are prime indications for…"?'

All in all, it becomes increasingly difficult to detect much difference between the technique of the prescriber and the vendor of drugs today, that of the witch doctor, or sharman, of old, who still practises in certain parts of the world, and that of the quack who has flourished all down the ages in the market places of Europe and North America. Not that it can be suggested for one moment that there were no fatalities, or near-fatalities, with the herbal remedies of old. Indeed, there must have been many an accident in these days of old when our forebears were experimenting with the effect of herbs in the curing, or alleviating, of disease. Superficially, or rather in theory, the patient of today is much better protected in this way by a mass of complicated legislation. What is responsible, at least in part, for the continuing high level of toxic effects from drugs is that our chemists, pharmacologists and doctors are becoming far too clever. They are producing and using powerful synthetic drugs aimed at acting on one particular part of the body, but finding again and again that they have a deleterious effect on some other part of the body.

It is this excessive tailoring of modern synthetic drugs, in order to get a maximum effect, that is making their administration so complicated and so risky that the unfortunate patient has to be under constant supervision. His blood pressure, for instance, may be brought down to a most satisfactory level, but he drops down in a faint on getting out of bed in the morning, or suddenly finds that he is dizzy boarding a bus or crossing a busy street. Here, for instance, is a list of the 'side-effects' of one currently widely-used drug: dizziness, blurring of vision, diarrhoea, depression, decrease of mental acuity, decreased libido, urticaria and eczema. With drugs obtained from herbs this risk of unwanted effects is often not as great, or at least can be more easily controlled.

There is also some evidence that in attempting to purify the active principle of a herb one of two things may happen. One is that it loses some or all of its potency. The other is that it becomes almost dangerously potent: it is as if there was some braking, or balancing, mechanism in the plant itself which prevented the active principle becoming too powerful. This is a point that is very much to the fore today with digitalis, the great stand-by in the treatment of the failing heart: this is fully discussed in chapter 2. It has also arisen, though to a lesser extent, in the case of rauwolfia, the tranquillizing and hypotensive (blood-pressure-lowering) drug we owe to India.

Even more fundamental, however, is the often ignored fact that the wisdom of the ages about herbs that heal has been acquired and accumulated over a long period. Today drugs come and go: here today, gone tomorrow. Seldom is there time to assess their value: some snag is found and out they go. Part of the trouble, of course, is our dependence on the pharmaceutical industry for new drugs, and the industry's complaint that it cannot exist profitably without producing a steady stream of new drugs. Indeed, their major complaint today is that it takes so long to get a new drug on to the market that it becomes increasingly difficult to make a viable profit. The result is the multiplicity of drugs, of which the Director-General of the World Health Organization complains, not the least important drawback of which is that doctors do not have time to study new drugs and their effect on their patients. Just as they are getting used to a new drug – understanding its mode of action, its side-effects and how it suits some patients, but not others – they are bombarded by a mass of high-powered propaganda from the pharmaceutical industry, urging them to drop this drug and start using another.

This may be good salesmanship, but it is bad medicine. The pharmaceutical industry has to realize that selling drugs does not lie in the same category as selling washing powders or motor cars. The profit-making basis of the pharmaceutical industry presents difficulties even to those to whom capitalism, with its profit-making basis, is the preferable form of society. Unfortunately, it is not a problem that the industry has ever faced up to in a thoroughly frank manner. This is not the place to discuss the practical problems, but it is to be hoped that the industry will be able to solve them.

One solution would be for the industry to give much more attention to the study and development of herbs that heal. As already indicated earlier in this chapter, this is an idea that is being broached, but much more needs to be done along these lines.

Rather than playing molecular roulette with synthetic substances in the hope that 'something will turn up', what is required is that the research worker should study herbs that are known to be effective in certain diseases, and with that information as a starting point, then proceed to synthesize modifications in the hope that they will be more effective than, or have a wider sphere of action than, the original herb. Already much useful information has been obtained in this way from a study of the effect of herbs in several diseases.

Incidentally, it is not irrelevant in this context to cast a passing glance at what is happening on the other side of the Iron Curtain. Hitherto the pharmaceutical industry on this side of the Curtain has claimed that much more progress has been made in the realm of new drugs in non-communist than in communist countries. To a certain extent this is true; but what is overlooked – intentionally or otherwise – is that to a large extent it has been the deliberate policy of Russia and her satellites to concentrate their pharmaceutical industry on the study of herbal remedies and to develop these whenever possible. It has further been a matter of policy that, when a satisfactory herbal remedy has been found and proved of value, then manufacturing concentrates on this, rather than on a multiplicity of new drugs following each other in quick succession, as in non-communist countries.

This is not the place to become involved in political arguments, but this concept of what has been described as 'exploiting folklore in herbal practice on a scientific basis' cannot have been a complete failure: for, as Professor E J Shellard pointed out in his inaugural lecture as Professor of Pharmacognosy at Chelsea College, University of London, today, all over the world, with perhaps the exception of Great Britain, a concentrated effort is being made, with financial backing from governments, to search the plant kingdom for new therapeutic agents, especially for those with anti-carcinogenic, anti-viral, anti-fertility and anti-fatigue properties.

Typical of this increasing interest in herbs that heal is the increasing number of national and international conferences being devoted to the subject. Thus, in 1974, the Pharmaceutical Society of Great Britain held a national conference on 'Herbal Remedies in Europe', while in 1975 it organized an international symposium on 'Secondary Plant Products of Commercial Importance'. In 1974, the International Pharmaceutical Federation included a medical plants section in its meeting in Rome; in 1975 there was an international conference on medical plants in Czechoslovakia; and a large portion of an international symposium on gerontology, in which the World Health Organization participated, was devoted to a discussion of the Chinese herbal preparation known as ginseng (see chapter 9).

But perhaps most interesting of all was the working party organized by the United Nations to discuss the problems being raised by the world shortage of opiates, which is manifesting itself in an acute fashion by a shortage of codeine, one of the most useful constituents of opium. This shortage cannot be met by the synthetic chemists, and the solution lies in producing larger amounts of thebaine which can be readily converted chemically to codeine. While found along with morphine in the poppy known as *Papaver somniferum*, the major source of medicinal opium, thebaine is present in much larger amounts in another poppy, *Papaver bracteatum*. The purpose of this working party, which was held in the USA, and attended by representatives from seventeen countries and twelve pharmaceutical companies, was to get down to the problem of how best to isolate the maximum amount of thebaine from this particular poppy. In other words, the first approach to the problem was by seeking the help of Nature – not the inmates of the research laboratory.

For a long time much play was made by critics of herbal remedies of the fuss that the old herbalists made about collecting herbs at some particular time of the day or year, or in relationship to the weather. This was held to be all hocus-pocus. How wrong these critics have proved to be! Research over the years has shown that, like good gardeners, these old herbalists were absolutely right and that the active principle of the plant, or herb, may vary considerably.

Thus, the yield of morphine from the poppy at 9 am is often four times the yield obtained twelve hours later. The same diurnal variation has been shown with various other plants, including atropine. In other cases the active principle varies with the stage of germination. Thus, in the case of the periwinkle (see chapter 3) there is virtually no active principle in the seeds. It appears during germination and by three weeks is present throughout the plant – only to disappear and then reappear at around eight weeks. Flowering often coincides with an increase in the active principle, but in some plants it decreases at this time. In other words the old herbalists knew what they were doing. They learned the hard way and the long way, whereas today, the application of modern techniques makes it possible to acquire this information more quickly.

Equally important is the variation in the constituents of the same plant, or species of the same genus, in different parts of the world. This was well brought home to the modern pharmaceutical industry in the case of rauwolfia and in the search for starting plant material for the manufacture of the sex hormones (see chapter 10).

No account of this herbal revolution would be complete without at least a passing reference to two of the best-known names in the field of herbal and what used to be known as patent medicines – not so much because of their fundamental contribution to the picture, fascinating though that was, but because they are representative of one of the biggest changes in this revolution.

Thomas Beecham I, as he would have been known in the USA,

world famous for his pills with their 'worth a guinea a box' slogan, was born in Oxfordshire in 1820. He started life as a shepherd boy but rapidly acquired a reputation locally as a herbalist. He quickly decided, however, that there was more money in so-called patent medicines, and it was in this sphere that he made his fortune.

Jesse Boot, later Lord Trent, was born thirty years later. His father was an ardent Wesleyan lay preacher and a keen advocate of the one belief shared by Wesleyans and Roman Catholics, namely that the Church was responsible for the body as well as the soul of man. By the nineteenth century the monastic tradition of healing may have been dying out in the Roman Catholic Church, but, under the active inspiration of John Wesley, it had permeated his followers. It was due to his father and his mother, particularly the latter in view of his father's death when he was only ten, that Jesse Boot became a herbalist – going out into the fields to collect his herbs. Soon, however, he realized that this was not the way to make the fortune he sought. It was much easier, and cheaper, to buy sacks of magnesium sulphate (Epsom salts) than to go trailing through the meadows collecting herbs that then required much attention before they were ready for sale. He, too, therefore gave up herbalism and blossomed out on the retailing side to take advantage of all the proprietary medicines that were then beginning to sweep the market. These may seem remote days to the younger generation, but it is of interest that it was only in 1975 that a member of the staff of Boots the Chemists, retired, whose uncle had been the fourth man to be taken on by Jesse Boot in his early days.

This loss of interest in herbs was not only due to the flood of 'patent medicines'; it also coincided with the initiation of the chemical era, when chemists were turning their new-found skills and knowledge to the synthesis of the active principles they were isolating from herbs. It was an era that expanded with increasing momentum, and by the turn of the century, particularly under the pressure of the German chemical industry, Nature's herbs were out and man-made drugs were in.

That ailing humanity benefited from these man-made drugs no-one will deny but, as usually happens with the scientist, he allowed his enthusiasm to run away with his sense of direction, and it was not until the discovery of penicillin that he began to turn back to Nature. This, incidentally, was a reversion that was encouraged by two factors. One was the alarming demonstration by Nature of her ability to counteract man-made drugs by inducing resistance to them. The other was the relative failure of the chemists to produce any effective anti-cancer drugs.

So today we are witnessing yet another swing of the pendulum: back to the herbs that heal. The century and more that has passed since Thomas Beecham gave up herbs for synthetic products has been an exciting and productive period, but there are good grounds for believing that the era which we are now entering will be just as exciting and productive. As Sir David Campbell said in 1930, during his inaugural lecture as Professor of Materia Medica in the University of Aberdeen: 'It is clear that faith in drugs, especially vegetable drugs, has been deep-seated and widespread amongst all peoples from the earliest times. It is as strong in modern civilization as it was amongst primitive man.'

It is to probe this persistent primeval faith, which has now come wellnigh full circle, that this book has been written, and to indicate at least some of the herbs that heal with which Nature so richly endows us.

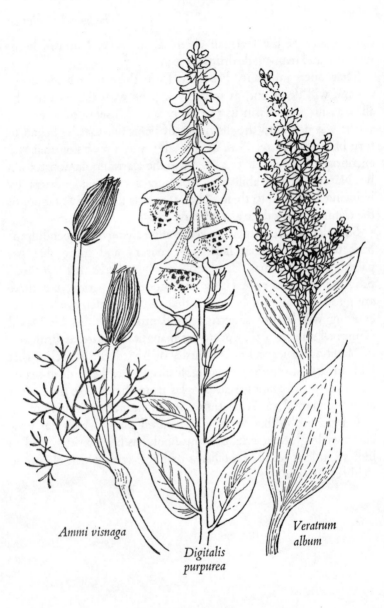

Ammi visnaga

Digitalis
purpurea

Veratrum
album

2
Herbs and the heart

Exactly 200 years have passed, as this chapter is being written, since a shrewd Birmingham physician made a casual observation that was to revolutionize the treatment of the failing heart and to be instrumental in prolonging the lives of millions of victims of heart disease.

The shrewd observer who made this casual observation and acted on it to the lasting benefit of ailing humanity, was William Withering, the son of an apothecary in Wellington, Salop. Born in 1741, he graduated MD from the University of Edinburgh in 1766, and the same year he was appointed one of the first two physicians to the newly opened Staffordshire Infirmary in Stafford.

He spent nine happy years in Stafford. Professionally they were not particularly busy ones as, in the case of the pre-National Health Service consultants, private patients tended to be few and far between in the early days of practice. One of the first of them, however – Helena Cooke, the seventeen-year-old daughter of the recently appointed town clerk of Stafford, and, according to Withering, a girl in whom 'the harpsichord, the voice, the pencil, and every exterior accomplishment were already at her command' – was, in due course, to become his wife. Not the least of these accomplishments, so far as her future husband was concerned, was her skill with the pencil, for Withering was using much of his spare time in preparing what was to become his first major work: *The Botanical Arrangement of all the Vegetables naturally growing in Great Britain*. Such a work obviously required accurate, attractive drawings, and it was by using Helena as artist that William had the opportunity of that regular association with her that finally, in 1772, was to blossom out into holy matrimony.

The compilation of the book coincided with his stay in Stafford. It was published in 1776, a few months after the Witherings moved to Birmingham, a move dictated largely by the fact that, as a married man, Withering began to realize that an annual income of around £100 (even allowing for some private income) was scarcely sufficient for a married man with domestic responsibilities. The book was an outstanding success, so much so that it was still going strong over a century later and the fourteenth edition appeared in 1877. In view of his subsequent masterpiece, and as an introduction to its history, the following excerpt from *The Botanical Arrangement* is of more than passing interest:

'Many people will be surprised to find so little said upon the medicinal virtues of plants, but those who are best enabled to judge of this matter will perhaps think that the greater part of that little might well have been omitted. The superstition of former years, operating upon the ignorance of mankind, gave rise to miracles of every denomination, and the fashion of combining a great variety of ingredients with a design to answer any particular purpose rendered the efficacy of any of them extremely doubtful. The dreadful apprehensions that men formerly entertained of poisons made them fearful of employing substances that were capable of doing mischief, and they therefore rejected those that were most likely to do good. A number of vegetables fit only for food were supposed to be capable of producing the greatest alterations in the human body, and at length every plant was esteemed a cure for almost every disease. In this situation of things little advantage can be reaped from the experience of former times. We shall sooner attain the end proposed if we take up the subject as altogether new, and, rejecting the fables of the ancient herbalist, build only upon the basis of accurate and well considered experiments.'

In other words, as Robert Burns was to express it, so far as Withering was concerned,

> 'But Facts are chiels that winna ding,
> An downa be disputed.'

Not for him were old wives' tales unless they could be supported by hard facts. Here he differed from both the free-wheeling herbalist on the one hand and the sceptical, hidebound medical profession on the other. His was the *via media*, which in this context might justifiably be described as the *vis medicatrix naturae*, the healing power of Nature. If Nature really does provide the means to overcome disease, then why not make full use of it? This brings us to the climax of his life: the publication in 1785 of *An Account of the Foxglove*, described nigh on two centuries later as 'the first scientific treatise on the treatment of disease written in English, and it remains today as one of the really great English contributions to treatment'.

As already mentioned, in 1775 Withering moved to Birmingham where, in due course, he was appointed one of the first physicians to the newly opened General Hospital. In order to help the Staffordshire Infirmary pending the appointment of a successor, Withering continued, for a while, to visit Stafford once a week. As this involved a journey of thirty miles each way, a change of horses was required en route. One day, while the change was being made, he was asked to see an old woman water-logged with dropsy. This he did, and decided that she was not long for this world. Some weeks later, he inquired how she was and, much to his surprise, learned that she had made a most satisfying recovery. This happy outcome, so different from his recent prognosis, intrigued Withering who asked if he might see her again. They met and she informed him that her recovery was due to a herbal tea she had taken.

And here let the tale be continued in Withering's own words.

'In the year 1775 my opinion was asked concerning a family receipt for the cure of dropsy. I was told that it had been kept a secret by an old woman in Shropshire, who had sometimes made cures after the more regular practitioners had failed. I was informed, also, that the effects produced were violent vomiting and purging, for the diuretic effects seemed to have been overlooked. This medicine was composed of twenty or more different herbs; but it was not very difficult for one conversant in these matters to perceive that the active herb could be no other than the foxglove.'

Thus began an investigation that was to culminate ten years later in the publication of *An Account of the Foxglove*, based upon the findings in 163 cases. Its significance as a milestone in the history of the treatment of disease can only be adequately assessed against the background of the then current status of the foxglove in the field of therapy. Known since the early years of the Christian era, it had had a variegated career at the hands of the herbalists. Its toxic potentialities were early recognized, and for this reason it was largely used as a salve or external application in the treatment of cuts, wounds and sores. On the age-old tradition that desperate conditions demand desperate remedies, it was also recommended for the treatment of epilepsy, but this was by no means a unique reason, as there can have been few herbs since the dawn of history that have not been commended at some time or another for this fear-inspiring and common condition. Its toxic potentialities were recognized by the fact that it was used as what the Americans so nicely describe as a 'chemical jury': in other words, its use in ordeal trials to determine whether or not an individual was guilty or innocent. If he survived he was innocent; if guilty, he died. As always down the ages to add a spice of variety to life, country folk took advantage of its poisonous attributes to produce a potent tea as a cheap means of intoxication.

In the course of time it achieved some reputation in the treatment of dropsy and chest conditions, including tuberculosis and asthma. Indeed, Withering studied its effect in tuberculosis but failed to obtain any evidence of a beneficial action. In spite of this, its anti-tuberculosis reputation persisted among doctors for many years after Withering's time. In fairness to them it has to be admitted that Withering rather sat on the fence, mainly because a Mr Saunders, an apothecary of Stourbridge, 'a man of repute and long experience' according to Withering, commended it highly for this purpose.

Its standing as a folk remedy in Withering's day is interestingly exemplified by the fact that it is mentioned in this capacity in George Eliot's *Silas Marner*, and in his book Withering himself records the story of the Yorkshire travelling tradesman, whom he was asked to see, whose wife had treated his asthma by stewing a large handful of foxglove leaves and giving him the resulting decoction. The unfortunate man was brought to death's door, with a pulse rate of forty, but fortunately he recovered. Withering commented, with characteristic conciseness: 'This good woman knew the medicine of her country but not the dose of it.'

What Withering so clearly showed in his *opus magnum* (207 pages plus coloured frontispiece. Price 5s.), was that preparations made from the purple foxglove (*Digitalis purpurea*, to give it its technical name) relieved dropsy due to certain forms of heart failure. As he remarked in a letter subsequent to the publication,

> 'Under my own management, under that of the medical practitioners of this part of England, and I may add, also in the hands of some worthy and respectable clergymen in village situations, it continued to be the most certain, and the least offensive diuretic we know in such cases, and in such constitutions as I have advised its exhibition.'

That this is no idle boast, but a plain statement of facts, is exemplified by the fact that nigh on two centuries of intensive investigation, clinical, biochemical and pharmacological, have added little to what Withering told us in his famous classic. His reason for its 'exhibition' is still the major indication – neglected, alas, all too often by the modern young heart specialist, convinced in his foolish arrogance that he can improve on Nature, and working through a computer and a laboratory rather than directly with the patient. Equally valid today is Withering's list of side-effects – still a salutary warning of the dangers of misusing a potent drug.

And a potent drug it is, as we have always known. It must therefore be treated with respect. If treated in this way, and used with circumspection, it is one of the most valuable drugs in the pharmacopoeias of the world. On the other hand, if abused or misused, as Withering pointed out, it can be unpleasantly dangerous. So much so, that only a few years ago a physician on the staff of one of the best teaching hospitals in the USA commented: 'The frequency and gravity of digitalis intoxication are not widely appreciated. Seldom a day elapses that we do not encounter either minor or major evidence of digitalis overdosage. Such experience has led a member of the house staff of the Peter Bent Brigham Hospital, Boston to remark that 'nowadays lanatoside [a preparation of digitalis] is replacing homicide as a leading cause of death'.

A less macabre example of the dangers of digitalis if not treated with respect is the tale told of Professor Purkinje, a distinguished nineteenth century Czech physiologist, whose main interest was the functioning of the brain. Having read that one of the side-effects of digitalis was the production of yellow vision, he decided to confirm this on himself. He therefore took enough digitalis to kill nine cats. The reason he chose this apparently esoteric method of measuring his dose is that the testing of the potency of a preparation of digitalis was worked out on cats, and this potency was measured in what became known as cat units. He soon bitterly regretted his decision for he vomited for a week, developed gross irregularity of heart action and experienced not inconsiderable heart pain. Fortunately he recovered – a wiser, if sadder, man.

But why has this valuable drug achieved this dire reputation? Mainly because too many doctors have given up using preparations of digitalis made from the entire leaf of the foxglove and have fallen for the advertising gimmicks of the pharmaceutical industry and are using the individual active constituents of the leaves, known as glycosides. One of the first impacts of the chemical and biochemical advances of last century on medicine was felt in materia medica, or pharmacology as it is now known – the study of drugs. The perfectly natural and justifiable aim here was to try and discover why drugs acted as they did, in the hope that, if the active constituents could be isolated, this might prove more effective than using the whole drug. This sometimes proved to be the case; in others it did not: digitalis proved to come in this latter category.

Digitalis was an obvious first target for the pharmacologists because it had always proved difficult to produce a standardized preparation of the leaves of the foxglove that would always have the same effect in a given dose. Equally worrying was the fact that certain preparations, such as the tincture, tended to go off quickly, even if kept in reasonable conditions. A further complication was that the margin between an effective dose and a toxic dose was relatively small. Logically therefore it appeared clear that the obvious line of attack was to isolate the active factors, or principles, in the foxglove leaf and hope that these would prove more amenable to standardization and have reasonable keeping properties. In due course the active glycosides were isolated. The pharmaceutical industry then cashed in and started producing a series of glycosides which they sold to doctors as the very last word in therapy.

As, unfortunately, all too often happens, doctors fell for this high-powered salesmanship – and not to the benefit of the patient. Undoubtedly some of these glycosides are useful and do not deteriorate over a period of time, but they are still as potentially dangerous as the preparations made from the whole leaf. What also needs to be stressed is that the official preparation of the *British Pharmacopoeia*, usually prescribed in tablet form, is equally effective for all practical purposes, and does not deteriorate in efficiency if kept in reasonable conditions. Not the least of the disadvantages of the digitalis glycosides now being so widely used is their very efficiency and the fact that they can be given by injection into the bloodstream, thus ensuring a quick action.

This, however, is frequently what is not required. To push digitalis to the maximum dose in order to get a quick response is asking for trouble. Slow and sure is the golden rule, working up to a dose that produces either the desired effect or incipient evidence of toxicity. This can be achieved as effectively, if not more so, by the use of the *British Pharmacopoeia* preparation known as digitalis leaf. So far as I am aware there is no convincing evidence that any of the individual glycosides in use today have any advantage over digitalis leaf, whether from the point of view of efficacy, toxicity or keeping properties. In parenthesis it may be added here that a recent survey of patients admitted to hospital with heart conditions treated by the most widely used of these digitalis glycosides showed that one in four was suffering from an overdose of the drug, and of these patients one in sixteen died of digitalis poisoning.

In other words, the attempt of the pharmaceutical industry to improve on Nature, and thereby increase their profits by trying to impose on doctors what it to claims be *the* active principle of the plant, has got us nowhere. Indeed, a case could well be made out for claiming that it has done more harm than good. By all means analyse a herb to discover its active principle, or principles, but let it never be forgotten that, in certain cases at least, the apparently active principle by itself may not be as active or as safe as a carefully prepared extract from the whole plant, or, in some instances, part of it, whether leaf, flower, rhizome, or root.

What is too often forgotten, however, is that digitalis is not the only drug of which the active principles have a specific action on the heart. Many plants are known to contain digitalis-like substances or glycosides. Indeed, one expert in this field has gone so far as to say that there must be something wrong with a philosophy which accepts what he describes as 'the dangerous *Digitalis purpurea*', but rejects the 'much safer' lily of the valley and completely ignores the 'extremely safe' hawthorn. Be the merits of these two herbs what they are (and they will be discussed briefly later in this chapter), there is one of the digitalis-like drugs – strophanthin – that is widely used in Europe.

There are two forms of strophanthin: one known as strophanthin-K and the other, more widely used one, as strophanthin-G (or ouabain). They have a fascinating history, of which that of strophanthin-K may be taken as an example. It comes from the dried seeds of *Strophanthus kombé*, a climbing plant indigenous to eastern tropical Africa, where it is used as an arrow poison. It came to the attention of David Livingstone in 1861, while he was exploring the Shire River, and he immediately realized its therapeutic value. Specimens were brought back to Kew Gardens, and in due course, in 1885, Professor T R Fraser, Professor of Materia Medica in the University of Edinburgh, isolated the active principle and named it strophanthin. This soon found its way into medical practice on account of its digitalis-like action and the fact that, unlike digitalis, it was active when given by intravenous injection. Strophanthin-G, or ouabain as it is officially known, is the active principle of *Strophanthus gratus*, which grows in West Africa and has a dire reputation locally as an ordeal poison. It is much more potent than strophanthin-K, and has the advantage that it contains a single principle, whereas strophanthin-K is a mixture of principles. This means that it can be more satisfactorily standardized and is therefore preferred today to strophanthin-K.

The great advantage of both of these is that they are active when given by intravenous injection. Two further advantages are that they do not have too prolonged an action and that they do not irritate the stomach as much as digitalis and are therefore less likely to cause sickness. In spite of the fact that one of the digitalis glycosides, digoxin, can also be given intravenously, experienced doctors prefer one of the strophanthin preparations if it is felt that a failing heart must be quickly brought under control. As has already been noted, such speed is not needed very often but, when it is, strophanthin is the answer – thus disposing of one of the arguments often put forward in favour of digoxin. In this context it is noteworthy that strophanthin-G is much more widely used in Europe than in the British Isles.

Two of the other plants that have a digitalis-like action, lily of the valley and hawthorn, have already been mentioned. It is of interest that preparations of lily of the valley are widely used in Russia for the treatment of heart conditions: yet another example of how the USSR prefers to use natural, rather than synthetic, drugs. Three other herbs are used by the Russians instead of digitalis. One of these is *Adonis vernalis*, or spring pheasant's eye, an anemone-like plant. Another is *Nerium oleandre*, from which a strophanthin-like principle, known as oleandrin, has been isolated and is included in the *Russian Pharmacopoeia*. The third is *Apocynum cannabinum*, a North American plant, also known as hemp dogbane, Indian hemp, and Canadian hemp, from which an active principle, known as cymarin, with a stro-phanthin-like action, has been isolated and is included in the *Russian Pharmacopoeia*. An interesting historical footnote to *Apocynum cannabinum* is that it was used with success to treat President Benjamin Harrison, the twenty-third President of the USA from 1889 to 1892, when he had a serious heart attack. Broom tops are an old popular remedy, dating back to Anglo-Saxon times for afflictions of the heart, a belief that modern re-search has shown to be justified, and to be due to an active principle known as sparteine.

There has been relatively little investigation into the many herbs recommended for the treatment of high blood pressure. Haw-thorn comes into this group as does mistletoe, which is still retained in the French and Spanish *Pharmacopoeias*, mainly for this purpose. Mistletoe, of course, has a reputation dating back to the Druids. Ever since, all down the ages, it has had a reputation as more or less an all-heal, having a beneficial effect on the heart, and also, curiously enough, on tumours, the application of the juice to a tumour being a well-recognized form of treatment. This is obviously a tradition (dating back, incidentally, to Pliny) which has not died out: the current edition of *The Extra Pharma-copoeia* (or *Martindale*, as it is often referred to after William Martindale, the compiler of the first edition in 1883), the wise doctor's therapeutic Bible, refers to a Swiss proprietary prepara-tion of mistletoe still on the market which is sold for use in cancer. Its use in high blood pressure dates back some seventy years, during which it has retained a fairly steady reputation in Europe.

I recall in the 1930s, Sir Maurice Cassidy, then one of the leading London heart specialists, telling me that several of the patients he had had referred to him on account of high blood pressure had been given mistletoe for its treatment in France. Being a wise physician he was not prepared to voice a definite opinion on its efficacy, though I gathered he was not sufficiently impressed with the results to put it on his prescribing list.

Of more proven value is green hellebore (*Veratrum viride*), also known as American hellebore, which has to be distinguished from black hellebore, or white Christmas rose, a plant indigenous to Europe, which has a digitalis-like action on the heart, but is seldom used for this purpose today. Green hellebore, a plant indigenous to North America, comes into quite a different category and has a long history of medical usage by the local Indians for a wide variety of conditions, including that of a heart tonic. Its use was taken up by the early settlers, but it did not penetrate to England until around 1860. In due course it was found to be similar in its properties to European, or white, hellebore (*Veratrum album*), but for a long time its major use was as an insecticide. It was not until the 1950s that it was found to contain active principles with a potent action in lowering the blood pressure and for a time it was widely used for this purpose. Today, partly because of the keen competition in the hypotensive (blood-pressure-lowering) market, it is somewhat under a cloud; but drugs wax and wane in popularity, just as do many other fashions, and green hellebore may well swing back into the hypotensive firmament.

Finally in this context, though not on the principle of keeping the best wine to the end, is the most important of all the blood-pressure-lowering herbs: rauwolfia – India's greatest contribution to modern therapy. In view of its versatility, however, its fascinating story is best told as a whole, and this is done in chapter 9.

Of all the afflictions of the heart, to which man is heir, perhaps the most dreaded is that known as angina pectoris. The dread is largely associated with the intense pain that is its presenting manifestation, and is due to narrowing of the coronary arteries which supply the blood to the heart. It is not always clear whether this narrowing is due to spasm or to thickening of the wall of the arteries, or to a combination of these two factors, but what is all too clear is that, if the heart muscle is deprived of an adequate supply of blood, then the result is excruciating pain with a typical distribution, whenever any movement is made. Few herbal remedies have been recommended for this condition, mainly because there is one drug, known as trinitrin, which is an almost infallible reliever of the pain.

In 1946, however, an article from Cairo appeared in the *British Heart Journal*. This drew attention to the value of a Middle-Eastern plant, known as *Ammi visnaga*, in the relief of the pain of angina pectoris. *Ammi visnaga*, known in Arabia as 'khella', grows wild in eastern Mediterranean countries, including the Nile delta, and in Arabia. From ancient times it has been used locally in folk medicine, especially for the relief of renal colic induced by stones in the kidneys. So well-established was this practice that a decoction of the seeds was often prescribed by the local doctors. Although the active principle, khellin, was isolated, albeit in a somewhat crude form, as long ago as 1879, it was not until the 1930s that Egyptian research workers began seriously to study the herb. This research showed that the plant brought relief by relaxing the spasm in the muscle fibres induced by stones in the kidneys or the ureters, the passages leading from the kidney to the bladder. As a result a tincture of *Ammi visnaga* was included in the *Egyptian Pharmacopoeia* in 1934.

Some ten years later Professor Anrep and his colleagues in Cairo University showed that khellin, now available in pure form, was a strong dilator of the coronary arteries. This immediately suggested that it might be of value in the treatment of angina pectoris and this was confirmed in their 1946 article, already mentioned, in which they reported favourable results in thirty-five out of thirty-eight patients with angina pectoris to whom they had given khellin. For various reasons, too technical to go into here, khellin never caught on in Britain, though it did gain official recognition in the French and Polish *Pharmacopoeias*. Be that as it may, it was an interesting demonstration of the rational basis which so often underlies the traditional use of herbal remedies. The fellaheen were absolutely right: their decoction of the seeds of *Ammi visnaga*, carefully harvested in 'the early morning as soon as the oldest flowers were ripe', did relieve the excruciating pain of what we know as renal colic, induced by stones – a much more common condition in the Middle East than in western Europe. The fact that it did not prove acceptable in Britain for the treatment of angina pectoris was merely incidental, and had nothing to do with the fact that here, as in the case of digitalis, was a herb that healed.

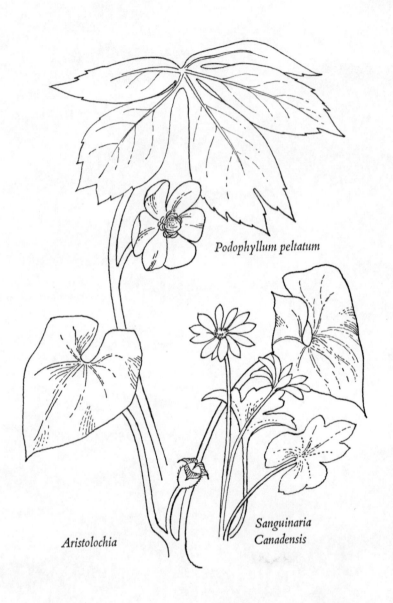

Podophyllum peltatum

Aristolochia

Sanguinaria
Canadensis

3

Herbs and cancer

During the last few months of his illness, when he was dying of cancer, Mr John Foster Dulles, the US Secretary of State, and his family, received some 600 unsolicited letters suggesting various forms of treatment for his cancer. Just over ten per cent of these recommended a range of herbal therapy, and fifty-seven plants were mentioned by name. These included two cactuses (one from Mexico and one from South Africa), St John's wort, creosote weed, garlic and the 'grape cure'. This last is a form of therapy which surfaces periodically on the wave of fashion or the more flamboyant outbursts of publicity-minded nations. One of its last resurrections was in the late 1960s when the Bulgarian Tourist Office linked the traditional longevity of Bulgarians with their country's superabundance of fruit, and recommended a series of 'special fruit cures' for a variety of illnesses. Among these was the 'grape cure', (three kilograms [six and a half pounds] a day once or twice a week), which was recommended for asthma, chronic bronchitis, and diseases of the liver and kidneys, with 'particularly good results' in 'patients suffering from exhaustion' – but with no mention of cancer.

This international gesture of goodwill for the dying Secretary of State epitomized – possibly in somewhat dramatic manner – the widespread belief that Nature had much to offer in the way of herbs that healed in cancer. It is a belief that dies hard, dating back, according to the experts, to at least the times of the Ebers papyrus (*circa* 1500 BC), in which herbal preparations are prescribed for what is thought to be cancer. The snag here, of course, is that as often as not it is impossible to be certain whether the swellings (for after all that is all that tumour means), said to disappear under the influence of a given herb were 'tumours', as we now recognize the term, far less a form of cancer. Even if they were tumours in our sense of the term, they may only have been the benign ones which we know to be amenable to treatment.

Another factor to bear in mind in this context is that for all practical purposes it was only superficial tumours, such as those of the breast or skin, that were recognized as such. More deep-seated tumours, such as those of the lungs, stomach and bowels, were almost certainly missed, and the patient diagnosed as suffering from 'cachexia' or some such vague condition. It is this blinkered outlook, literally and metaphorically, that also explains why so many of the quack cancer remedies, of which we heard so much until the advertising of such remedies was banned in quite recent times, were what are known as escharotics: that is, caustic or corrosive substances that 'burned' the tumour out. With a benign tumour, or that type of cancer of the skin that is localized to one spot, this may be quite an effective, if painful and deforming, way of getting rid of it. If, however, the tumour was a cancerous one, as in the breast, which had already spread elsewhere, the results were tragically catastrophic – all too often a literal hell on earth for the unfortunate victim.

It is against this background that any comments about the drug treatment of cancer must be viewed, and any attempt made to assess the claims that have come down to us from the past and are still found in the more backward parts of the world. But the fact that one must have a particularly ample supply of grains of salt does not detract from the interest – indeed, the fascination – of this age-old search for herbs that heal cancer.

Of the many herbs recommended in this sphere, only one or two will be mentioned before passing to a more detailed consideration of three that really have proved of value. Of the 'also rans', two are mentioned in other chapters: mistletoe and garlic. The use of mistletoe for this purpose dates back at least to ancient Rome, when it was recommended by Pliny the Elder (AD 23–79), and there is some experimental evidence that it has an inhibitory effect on certain tumours in mice. Unfortunately, this is not backed up by any valid evidence of its value in human cancer. In this field garlic has an equally ancient pedigree, dating back to the Ebers papyrus, which refers to its external application for 'indurations'. Hippocrates (*circa* 470–400 BC), who was no lover of drugs, mentions it for the treatment of tumours of the uterus, and a millennium later Indians were claiming that it cured abdominal tumours. And so it goes on, right down to the present day when it is said that in France the incidence of cancer is lowest where the consumption of garlic is highest, while in Bulgaria garlic eaters are said not to develop cancer. The New World is not immune from the anti-cancer reputation of this odoriferous herb, and in Texas and California it possessed for a long time, and probably still does, a folk-lore reputation for the treatment of cancer of the lungs and leukaemia. Even in the laboratory there is some evidence that concentrated garlic juice can arrest the growth of certain experimentally induced tumours in animals.

Plants of the *Euphorbiaceae* family also have an anti-tumour reputation dating back to Hippocratic days, and recent reports from the USA suggest that these claims may have a scientific justification. Research workers in the Department of Chemistry at the University of Virginia, Charlottesville, have isolated a substance which is active against leukaemia in mice from two members of this family, *Euphorbia escula* and *Croton tiglium. E. escula* is the well-known house plant, while *C. tiglium* is the source of croton oil, a violent purgative, a drop of which on a lump of sugar was a favourite purge in our grandparents' time.

The fact that these two plants contain substances which are active against leukaemia in mice by no means guarantees that they will be effective in the treatment of leukaemia in human beings. Too often in the past false hopes based on such findings have been dashed to the ground, but a careful study of the chemical structure of these substances may well give a useful clue to the chemical structure of a really potent anti-leukaemia drug.

Another of these traditional herbal cures for cancer is blood-wort, or *Sanguinaria canadensis*, a plant indigenous to Canada and the northern part of the USA. It contains several alkaloids and a red resin which is used by the Cherokee Indians as the source of a red dye to paint themselves. They also used a preparation of the plant for treating cancer of the breast, a practice that was taken up in a big way in the last century by the cancer quacks who throve in the USA. It even gained the notice of orthodox doctors, one of whom, a Dr Fell, produced, in 1857, a salve of which it was an active constituent, which became well enough known to achieve a trial at the Middlesex Hospital in London, but with contradictory results. On a more cautious plane it became quite popular for the treatment of warts and of polypi in the nose. Two of its alkaloids have been shown to exert what has been described as 'a notable therapeutic action on Ehrlich carcinoma in mice' and 'a significant necrotizing effect on sarcoma–37 in mice'. So, once again, there is some scientific evidence for its folklore reputation but, unfortunately, not sufficient to justify its use in the treatment of human cancer.

Of all the herbs in this category, perhaps the most curious, not so much on account of their anti-cancer properties as of the variegated claims that have been made for them in other branches of medicine, are several species of *Aristolochia*. The best known are the two named, respectively, Texan and Virginian snakewort. These names they acquired from their reputation in the treatment of snake bites, a reputation that, interestingly enough, is almost universal, being attached to different species found in South America and Africa. The Texan and Virginian varieties, known as serpentary, were introduced into England from North America in the seventeenth century, being admitted to the *London Pharmacopoeia* in 1650, with a mixed bag of indications, including principally that of a general stimulant and tonic. Latterly its more decorous recommendation was as a bitter, and it only finally disappeared from the *British Pharmaceutical Codex* some twenty years ago.

The name, *Aristolochia*, is from the Greek and means 'best birth'. This name was soon converted to birthwort, by which several species are known, including the species which grows in India (Indian *Aristolochia*, or Indian birthwort), and one which was originally introduced to Britain from central and southern Europe. It owes its name to one of the old herbal traditions: that known as the doctrine of signatures. According to this, the indications for the medicinal use of a plant depended on its shape. Thus, if it was kidney shaped it would be good for diseases of the kidneys. In the case of *Aristolochia* its resemblance to the uterus gave it its obstetric reputation. While it was chiefly used to encourage conception and aid childbirth, it was equally valued, apparently, for 'controlling menstruation' and inducing abortion.

One of the traditional uses of Indian *Aristolochia* was in the treatment of chronic skin ulcers. As the probability was that some at least of these were cancerous, some twenty years ago research workers at Wisconsin University decided to screen it for anti-tumour activity. This decision was enhanced by their finding that extracts of various species of *Aristolochia* had been used for the treatment of cancer in a practice going right back to the Graeco-Roman period. They therefore obtained a supply of the plant from Madras, and isolated from the roots a substance which they named aristolochic acid. This they found to be active against an experimental tumour in mice known as adenocarcinoma 755. In due course it was tried out on twenty patients with advanced cancer but, in the words of the report on this trial,

> 'no significant tumour regression was seen; several patients had transient relief of pain' but 'the renal toxicity of this drug was prohibitive ... Because the compound had no demonstrable anti-tumour effect in this small series of patients further exploration of dosage was not considered worth the risk ...'

But there was an unexpected sequel arising out of this renal toxicity. In the early 1960s a new form of fatal kidney disease appeared in the Danube basin in some ten restricted areas of Yugoslavia, Romania and Bulgaria. In some villages over one in ten of the inhabitants were stricken with Balkan nephropathy, as it was named, half the cases dying within two years. In Bulgaria alone, between 1961 and 1970, 1546 cases were diagnosed, 663 of which proved fatal. The search for the cause continues. It may be a virus but one possible culprit is *Aristolochia clematis*, or birthwort, which grows freely in the affected areas, competing successfully with wheat and other grain crops in certain soils. The experts differ, some contending that birthwort is unevenly distributed in the affected areas and that it is difficult to envisage how the toxin could be incorporated in foodstuffs except by design. On the other hand, there is the well-proved evidence of how toxic birthwort can be to the kidneys by virtue of the aristolochic acid it contains, and the relatively widespread distribution of the plant in the afflicted regions.

And so to the three herbs that stand out as welcome indicators of what may be awaiting the patient researcher in this field of cancer therapy. In order of increasing importance, and the sequence in which they will be dealt with (on the principle of keeping the best wine to the end), they are podophyllum, colchicum and the periwinkle.

Two species of podophyllum are included in the *British Pharmaceutical Codex: Podophyllum peltatum*, also known as American mandrake and may apple, and *Podophyllum emodi* or Indian podophyllum. The former is common in moist, shady sites in the eastern USA and eastern Canada, while the latter flourishes in the temperate forests of the lower slopes of the Himalayas. For all practical purposes they are comparable in their actions, and both have a long medical history, dating back in the case of the Indian plant to the early days of Hindu civilization. The active constituents, both present in the resin produced from the plant, which is included in the *British Pharmacopoeia*, are highly irritant. They are responsible for the plant's original claim to orthodox medical fame – as the virulent purgative so beloved by Victorian doctors as an antidote for the over-eating and over-drinking of so many of their patients. In this they were following the tradition of the American Indians among whom it was used as a purgative, as an emetic to induce vomiting, and for the treatment of worm infestations.

It was also used as a cancer cure by the Penobscot Indians of Maine. This aroused the interest of Dr J L Hartwell, of the US Cancer Chemotherapy Centre. Writing in 1960, he reported that he had letters on his files relating to the current use of an extract of the root in the treatment of leukaemia in Ohio, and of cancer in Virginia, and of an ointment made from the root for 'the removal of tumourous growths from livestock' in Indiana. He also found that in Lousiana an extract of the root had been a popular remedy for venereal warts for many years. These last two uses link up with the cauterizing, or escharotic, properties of podophyllum which today have been officially recognized by the use of podo-phyllum resin in the treatment of genital, or venereal, warts. It has also been used in the treatment of cancer of the skin.

Unfortunately its use for genital warts seems to be its only useful contribution to medicine, although experimentally it has been found active against tumours in mice. A Swiss pharma-ceutical company has also isolated an anti-cancer agent by partial synthesis: this got as far as a clinical trial in patients with cancer of the breast and the digestive tract, but the results were not gratifying enough to justify its further use.

In moving to colchicum we are getting hotter in our search for a genuine anti-cancer herb. The genus takes its name from Colchis in Asia Minor, where it has thrived for centuries. The species used medicinally is *Colchicum autumnale*, also known as meadow saffron and autumn crocus, though it has nothing to do with saffron and is not a crocus, but a member of the lily family. It likes moist, rich meadow land and grows abundantly in Gloucestershire, Worcestershire, Hampshire, Oxfordshire and Warwickshire, but commercially supplies come from Poland, Czechoslovakia, Yugoslavia and the Netherlands. In parts of England its local name is naked boys – as the flowers appear without leaves.

It had a high reputation among the Byzantine physicians of the fifth century for the treatment of joint conditions, but its history goes much further back, as the Ebers papyrus of *circa* 1500 BC records the prescription of colchicum and describes arthritis in the great toe. Theophrastus (380–286 BC), the father of botany, is said to be responsible for one of its many names, ephemera, signifying that anyone who took it would not live more than one day. Legendary though this tale may be, it typifies the re-spect, amounting almost to dread, in which colchicum was held by the ancients on account of its toxicity, and in spite of the fact that the Arab physicians recommended its use for gout, it was not until the late eighteenth century that it became at all widely used: this was on the recommendation of Baron Anton von Stock, physician to the Empress Maria Theresa, for the alleviation of dropsy. Its reincarnation as the sovereign remedy for gout we owe to Husson, a French army officer, whose secret remedy, 'Eau Médecinale', containing colchicum, achieved popularity in the reign of Louis XV. It was an Ipswich doctor, Dr W H Williams, who was responsible for its popularization as a gout remedy in England, with its inclusion in the *Pharmacopoeia* in 1824. Benjamin Franklin is reputed to have introduced it into North America.

It still stands supreme as an alleviator of the pain of acute gout, used in the form of the active principle, colchicine, which was first isolated in 1820. It was almost as an incidental finding in the course of studying its action in gout that it was discovered that it had what is known as an anti-mitotic action: that is, it arrested the growth of young cells. As this effect seemed to be particularly potent in the case of the white blood cells, the possibility immediately arose of its use in the treatment of leukaemia, the condition characterized by uncontrolled overproduction of these white blood cells. This supposition proved correct, and in the form of colchicine, or another alkaloid, demecolcine, it turned out to be one of the first drugs effective in bringing this dreaded disease under control. It proved valuable in the most killing of all the forms of leukaemia – the acute form. Today it has been largely replaced by other drugs, though the current edition of the major British textbook of paediatrics still lists it as one of 'the nine different anti-leukaemic drugs of established value in childhood acute lymphoblastic leukaemia'.

Here then is a herb that really alleviates, though it may not heal, cancer. For a really potent herb in this context (and the climax of this chapter) we have to turn to *Vinca rosea*, or *Catharanthus roseus* as the experts insist it should be named, but probably best known as that charming decorative shrub, the periwinkle. It has a long and ancient history dating back to Graeco-Roman days, and tinged with the almost inevitable mixture of superstition and practice. Thus, Nicholas Culpeper, in his famous *The Complete Herbal*, published according to his introduction, 'from my house in Spitalfields, next door to The Red Lion 5th September 1653', records that 'Venus owns the herb, and saith, that the leaves eaten by man and wife together cause love between them'. On a less exotic, or erotic, level is its reputation as a healer of piles and ulcerated skin, while chewing it was said to relieve toothache. Roger Bacon is quoted as claiming that bands of periwinkle stem tied round a limb relieved, or even prevented, cramp.

Today, however, its herbal reputation rests upon its claimed efficiency in treating diabetes: so much so that, according to a recently published book on herbs, 'today it is the accepted treatment of herbalists for diabetes'. This is a reputation it enjoys in all five continents: in England, Queensland, South Africa (among both Whites and Bantus), the Philippines, and in the West Indies, especially Jamaica and the Grenadines. It was this reputation for treating diabetes that led to the two-pronged investigation of it that culminated in the discovery of its hitherto unsuspected anti-tumour activity.

The story starts in 1949 when Professor R L Noble, then working in the Collip Medical Research Laboratory in the University of Western Ontario, London, Ontario, was investigating what he himself described as 'various plant extracts to which historical hearsay had ascribed empirical uses by primitive peoples'. In the course of his studies he learned of a bush tea used in the West Indies which was supposedly useful in diabetes. This interested him as he was primarily an endocrinologist with a special interest in insulin, the hormone produced by the pancreas which controls the metabolism of sugar in the body, and the lack of which induces the condition we know as diabetes mellitus.

He therefore obtained a supply of the plant from which this particular bush tea was made, and which turned out to be *Vinca rosea*: he tried it out in rabbits, but obtained no lowering in the level of sugar in the blood, which he should if the herb was to be of any use in controlling diabetes. And there the story might well have ended had not Professor Noble's interest in the periwinkle been renewed by stories of a periwinkle proprietary preparation having been marketed in England for some time for the treatment of diabetes. He therefore decided to have another shot at it, this time injecting the extract of the herb into rats, whereas in his first investigation he had given it by mouth to rabbits.

This time things did happen – though not exactly according to expectations. Within a week, practically all the injected rats had died of a roaring septicaemia. An investigation was immediately set afoot to find out why such an apparently disgraceful thing should have happened in a well-run modern research institute, and in due course the explanation was found. The rats died of this overwhelming infection, not because of any carelessness on the part of the operators, but because the periwinkle extract had knocked out and killed all the white blood cells in the rats' bodies, which normally protect them – as they do human beings – against infection. Without these protective white cells, the least infection can run riot in the body and produce a fatal result.

This immediately suggested the possibility that the periwinkle might be of value in the treatment of leukaemia which (as already mentioned in discussing colchicum) is characterized by uncontrolled over-production of such cells. Or, in the scientific language of Dr C T Beer, who was then working with Professor Noble on this project with a grant from the British Empire Cancer Campaign: 'Since substances capable of limiting the white cell population may have potential therapeutic value in the treatment of leukaemia, the isolation of the active principle was considered worthwhile'.

Such proved to be the case and in 1958 Professor Noble was able to report to the New York Academy of Sciences that he and his colleagues had isolated an active principle, or alkaloid, adding, with characteristic caution: 'Limited investigation for carcinostatic activity has been made from time to time as material was available. The crude material possessed some definite carcinostatic activity against transplantable mammary adenocarcinoma in mice and against a transplantable sarcoma in the rat.'

It is at this stage of one of the most exciting stories in the recent history of medicine that the second prong appears. This was Dr Gordon H Svoboda who, Professor Noble learned at the symposium in which he read his paper, had been working along the same lines and had reached the same conclusions: that the periwinkle was not worth following up as a remedy for diabetes, but that it held quite high possibilities as an anti-tumour agent. Dr Svoboda's interest in the periwinkle had been first aroused because he was on the research staff of Eli Lilly, the major producers of insulin in the USA. Having heard that during the 1939–45 War diabetics in the Philippines had used a local herb when they were cut off from supplies of insulin, he decided to investigate the plant, which turned out to be a local species of periwinkle.

The obvious sequel was that the two lines of investigation should be combined, and such was the case with most satisfying, if somewhat staggering, results. The staggering result is that nearly ninety alkaloids have now been isolated from different species of *Vinca*, and the poor old periwinkle has become so scientifically important that in 1974, a USA publisher felt justified in issuing a $32 monograph on the subject. At one time, too, it looked as if supplies of the periwinkle might run out, but fortunately extensive horticultural work in Hungary is producing adequate amounts at an economical rate.

Fortunately, this plethora of research has not held up the good work of applying the fruits of this investigation to the alleviation of suffering humanity. Two of these alkaloids – vinblastine and vincristine – are now in the *British Pharmaceutical Codex*, and proving of value in the treatment of a variety of malignant conditions. Indeed, such a useful role are these products of the periwinkle playing in the chemotherapy of cancer that they are both included among the first choices for the treatment of a range of different forms of tumour growth. And all because some doctors were percipient enough to realize that Nature provides herbs that heal.

But on this occasion I propose to leave the last word with two prominent American workers in the field of the chemotherapy of cancer, one writing in 1962 and the other a decade later. My 1962 quotation is:

'Before we condemn too harshly these ancient empirical, if not unscientific, attempts at cancer chemotherapy we should be reminded that at least 3% of over 1,500 plant extracts or plant products screened by the National Cancer Institute showed anti-tumour activity against one or more transplantable mice tumours. It is easy to ridicule medieval recipes; it is more difficult and may be wiser to investigate them.'

My 1972 quotation is:

'Recent studies in the isolation and structural elucidation of tumour inhibitors of plant origin are yielding a fascinating array of novel types of growth-inhibitory compounds. There appears to be reason for confidence that this approach may point the way to useful templates [moulds] for new synthetic approaches to cancer chemotherapy.'

When it is realized that in the last decade around 75,000 different plant species have been systematically screened in the USA for anti-tumour activity, it will be appreciated how, on that side of the Atlantic at least, a determined effort is at long last being made to discover what Nature has to provide in helping us to bring cancer under control.

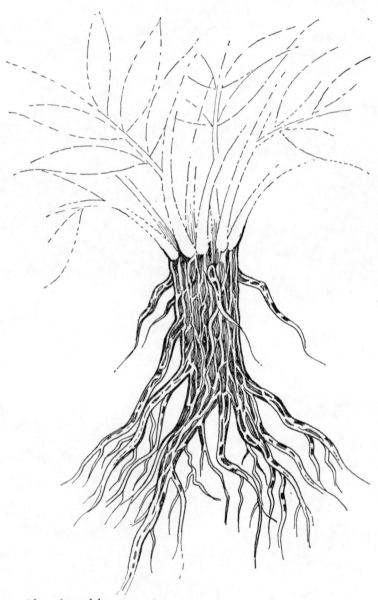

Glycyrrhiza glabra var. typica

4

The liquorice story

During the 1939–45 War an observant Dutchman, Dr F E Revers, noticed that some of his patients with peptic ulcer were doing particularly well. On questioning them he found that they had one feature in common – they were all taking a preparation supplied by a local pharmacist. Instead of turning up his nose at such unqualified practice, he decided to look into the matter, and found that the preparation contained the equivalent of 40% of powdered liquorice extract. Why liquorice should prove beneficial in the treatment of gastric ulcer was one of the mysteries of life that his textbooks did not explain but, having the curiosity of the born naturalist, which every good family doctor is, he decided to try it out by prescribing it for his patients afflicted in this way – and with excellent results.

Unfortunately he ran into the snag of so much modern treatment with drugs, namely, side-effects, and some of these were quite disconcerting as they included high blood pressure and dropsy. He was not to be put off, however. He had got the bit between his teeth and he was determined to get to the bottom of the mystery, having first reassured himself that the side-effects could easily be arrested by withdrawing the administration of liquorice. The upshot was one of the most important discoveries in modern therapy: namely, that liquorice has a cortisone-like action and that, in the words of one of the most experienced workers in this field, it is 'one of the most significant contributions to the treatment of gastric ulcer for fifty years'. Another expert in this field has stated that the synthesized derivative of liquorice that is now used for this purpose is:

'The first drug which convincingly has been shown to accelerate the healing of chronic gastric ulcer. To say that it melts away ulcers would be an exaggeration. To say that it considerably facilitates the healing process and enables patients to be treated as outpatients and not in hospital, is a fair comment.'

That was in 1968. Seven years later he was able to add:

'Over the years there has been a long succession of claims made for facilitating healing of gastric ulcer, but so far, apart from carbenoxolone [as this liquorice derivative is known] none has survived the test of time.'

Would that there were more such doctors as this Dutch one in our midst today: men and women with the curiosity of the born naturalist who, like Dr Withering (the discoverer of digitalis, the heart drug) and Dr Revers, have an observant eye and insatiable curiosity which, combined with a searching mind, are the basis of good doctoring and good research.

To appreciate the tremendous stride represented by this promotion of the liquorice all-sorts of our childhood days to one of today's really valuable drugs, a glance back over the history of liquorice will provide a salutary lesson and a useful reminder that, as in all aspects of human activity, the history of mankind must never be neglected. So far as liquorice is concerned, it is a long glance back. For three millenniums it has been used by mankind, one of the earliest records of it being in early Assyrian tablets. It is also listed in the papyri of ancient Egypt. Since then it has been used by civilization after civilization – Sumerians, Babylonians, Hindus, Chinese, Greeks and Romans – right down to the present day.

Theophrastus, who was named by Aristotle as his successor in the presidency of the Lyceum at Athens, writes in his *Enquiry into Plants*, which described some 500 plants, that 'Scythian root', as it was known by some:

'Is also sweet. Some call it simply sweet root. It is useful against asthma and in several troubles of the chest and also administered in honey for wounds. It has the property of quenching thirst, wherefore they say that the Scythians with this and mares'-milk cheese can go eleven to twelve days without drinking.'

The Romans thought so highly of it that it was included in the rations of the Roman legions.

Its use in Britain dates back to at least the thirteenth century, as it is mentioned in the accounts of Henry III, and both Chaucer and Shakespeare refer to it. Its traditional association with Pontefract dates back to the sixteenth century, when the Black Friars are said to have started growing it there. For long it throve here, bringing Pontefract national fame as the home of the Pontefract cakes, or little black lozenges of liquorice, that were the precursors of that still popular confectionery – liquorice all-sorts. Alas, the liquorice groves of Pontefract have fallen on evil days, but an attempt is now being made to revive them in view of the current increase in demand. The hard fact of life, however, is that the harvesting of liquorice is a back-breaking job, which no one has been able to mechanize and in these days of the pseudo-welfare state back-breaking jobs are not allowed by those who govern us – whether in Whitehall or in the marble halls of the mighty trade unions. We have therefore become dependent for our liquorice on those countries – on both sides of the Iron Curtain – in which hard manual labour is still part and parcel of the way of life. As a footnote to this historical survey, it is of interest that Napoleon's valet reported that Bonaparte had a weakness for his liquorice pellets.

Liquorice, or *Glycyrrhiza* to give it its botanical name, thrives in many parts of the world, with a predilection for river valleys with deep, sandy but fertile soil. There are several species of it, but the most satisfactory from the medicinal point of view – *Glycyrrhiza glabra* var. *typica* – is a plant four to five feet high, with purple-bluish flowers, and deep penetrating roots which possess long runners up to six feet long. Hence the difficulty in harvesting it, already mentioned, as it is the root that contains the essential medicinal ingredients. It is cultivated in Spain (in Old Castile, Navarra, Aragon, Catalonia, Valencia and Andalusia), Italy (in Calabria and Sicily), France, Germany and the USA (in Louisiana and California). Of the other species, one flourishes wild in the valley of the Volga, producing the so-called Russian liquorice, and another in the valley of the Tigris and Euphrates, yielding the so-called Persian liquorice, as much of it comes from Iran. There is yet another species which grows in Manchuria, and is known as Manchurian liquorice. This differs from other species in having relatively little sugar in the root and producing an unpleasantly pungent extract.

The important constituent of liquorice root is glycyrrhizin, which is about fifty times sweeter than cane sugar. It is to this that liquorice owes its sweet taste which for long dictated one of its main uses in orthodox medicine: namely, to disguise the taste of nauseating medicines. Down the ages, however, it has had a much more variegated career.

The Chinese, with what one might almost describe as their

traditional vested interest in longevity, valued it as a rejuvenator. More widespread was its use as a demulcent, or soother, particularly for congested throats and lungs. Hence its use in the treatment of lung troubles, to soothe a dry, hacking cough, and as an expectorant to help to bring up the sputum. For this soothing action there is a sound basis as liquorice contains what are known as saponins. These are natural substances which have a detergent-like action and therefore help to break up and loosen the mucus in the air passages which is responsible for much of the cough in infections of the throat and lungs. Liquorice also had a reputation for having a soothing action on the alimentary tract, whether the stomach or the bowel, and also of being a mild laxative. In the days when our forebears did not have quite the same respect for their innards as we have, partaking of gargantuan amounts of indigestible, highly spiced, often contaminated food, washed down by fantastic amounts of alcoholic liquor, this reputation as a soother of the insulted gut, or, as one old herbal puts it, 'a protection against the acrimony of food', was a valuable selling point. There may well be other factors involved in this healing effect on the gut, which will be discussed more relevantly later in this chapter when we consider the role of liquorice in the treatment of gastric ulcer.

Two other common uses of liquorice in medicine may also be mentioned. One is a common practice in France: its use as an eye lotion for the treatment of inflamed eyelids. This use has been taken up by the Chinese who have reported satisfactory results from the use of eye-drops containing sodium salts of glycyrrhinic acid, one of the active constituents of liquorice root, in the treatment of inflammation of the firm membrane that covers the eyeball. The interest of this revival of an old folklore use of liquorice is that the modern treatment of this particular affliction of the eye consists in part of the use of eye-drops containing some cortisone-like substance. As we now know that liquorice has a cortisone-like action, is this another example of modern science providing justification of traditional methods of treatment? Equally interesting in this context is its use to promote healing of the socket after dental extraction.

The same possibility arises with regard to its use in the treatment of certain skin diseases. This was a method that was re-introduced in the 1950s following the discovery of the cortisone-like action of liquorice. At the moment it has fallen into disuse, largely because the experts could not agree on its value, and when the experts – at least the medical ones – disagree in public, it is difficult for truth to penetrate the haze of battle. On this occasion, however, the probable explanation is that different people were using different concentrations of the active principle. Be that as it may, the noise of battle has quietened, but it would not be sur-prising if one of these days an up and coming young dermato-logist surfaces with the 'discovery' that liquorice is good, for example, for psoriasis.

Before considering the supreme role which liquorice now occupies in the treatment of gastric ulcer, and to complete the picture of the range of action of this versatile plant, its five non-medical uses must be mentioned. Prominent among these is its use in the tobacco industry, particularly in the USA where some pipe tobaccos contain up to 10% of liquorice. To many smokers this is an acquired taste, but to others it improves both the flavour and the smoking quality of the tobacco. This, of course, is why it is cultivated to such an extent in the USA. There is also a con-siderable amount used in snuff. Another major user is the con-fectionary trade, where it seems to retain its popularity with succeeding generations of children, if not their more sophisticated parents. What is left over after the essentials have been extracted is used in three other non-medical products: fire extinguishers, the manufacture of insulating mill board, and as mushroom compost. What more could one demand of one plant?

The story of the stomach (or gastric) healing properties of liquorice is such a typical example of what can be achieved by the careful study of folklore medicine that it is well worth telling in some detail. Actually it dates back practically seven decades to 1907, when what we now know to be the active principle, glycyrrhizin, was first isolated by Professor Alexander Tschirch in the pure crystalline state. This is a white crystalline powder, which gives the characteristic bitter-sweet taste of liquorice. No-one, however, attached any great significance to it, and it lay fallow in the dusty records of pharmacology for nigh on forty years.

In this long delayed period of recognition, curiously enough, it met the same fate as sulphanilamide, the first of the sulphonamide drugs. This was first isolated in 1908, but it was not until 1932 that Gerhard Domagk first spotted its antibacterial properties – described by a well-known British bacteriologist as 'the greatest advance ever made in chemotherapy'. The discovery of the healing properties of glycyrrhizin may not rank quite as high in the hierarchy of drugs, but it is of more than passing interest that two such valuable drugs should have been so long on the shelf before their therapeutic potentialities were realized. In the case of sulphanilamide the problem is particularly intriguing because on at least two occasions between 1908 and 1932 (1913 and 1919) reports were published indicating that this chemical structure was associated with antibacterial activity. Yet nothing happened until, almost incidentally, Domagk and his colleagues stumbled on the possibilities, with the resulting publication on Christmas Day, 1932, of the first German patent for 'prontosil' as the progenitor of sulphanilamide was known. It could be argued that the same thing applied to penicillin, but here there is what one might describe as a logical, or rational, explanation for the twelve-year gap. When Sir Alexander Fleming discovered penicillin in 1928 he realized its potentialities, but biochemistry had not the 'know-how' to isolate penicillin in sufficiently pure form to make it a feasible proposition. Indeed, neither would Lord Florey and his colleagues in Oxford have been able to do this had it not been for the exigencies of war overcoming the financial costs which would have precluded any pharmaceutical company under-taking on its own the initially difficult, elaborate and expensive fermentation process for its production.

In the case of liquorice perhaps there is more excuse for the delay in associating glycyrrhizin with the traditional healing properties of the plant. Its isolation coincided with the advent of science into medicine. The so-called 'wise men' were acquiring a snobbish disdain for folklore medicine, and the wisdom of the ages was barred from the ivory towers in which medical research was becoming enmeshed. The result was a blinkered outlook on life: nothing outside the walls of the laboratory was of any significance, and the doctor inside the laboratory never felt it necessary to consult the doctor at the bedside – unless, and until, in a somewhat lordly manner, he presented him with what he considered to be a useful drug.

So it befell that glycyrrhizin was ignored until the clinical antennae of a Dutch doctor, trained in the best tradition of clinical observation, detected the possible implications of his pharmacist neighbour's treatment for gastric ulcer. As mentioned earlier in this chapter, Dr Revers soon produced convincing evidence that this healing effect was due to the liquorice in the preparation. His initial elation was soon modified when he found that the healing process was complicated by undesirable effects such as oedema (or dropsy), high blood pressure, headache, dizziness, tightness in the chest and shortness of breath: obviously a price not worth paying for the healing of the offending ulcer in the stomach. Fortunately, withdrawal of liquorice banished these side-effects, and in many patients it was possible to attain at least a certain degree of healing of the ulcer by a dose of liquorice that produced no undesirable effects.

By a happy coincidence it was around this period (1949) that Dr Philip Hench and his colleagues at the Mayo Clinic, Rochester, Minnesota, announced the dramatic effect of cortisone on the course of rheumatoid arthritis. The whole medical world, clinical and scientific, was therefore agog with excitement and working overtime in studying the action of cortisone and comparable hormones. When therefore it was discovered that the oedema induced by liquorice was due to the retention in the body of sodium and chloride ions, and an excessive excretion of potassium ions from the body, this was immediately linked with the exactly comparable action of a hormone known as deoxycortone (or DOCA for short), which is one of the main constituents of the suprarenal glands. These glands (there are two of them – one on either side perched on top of the kidneys) are essential for life and when, as in the condition known as Addison's disease, they are destroyed by disease, then death is inevitable. At least it was inevitable until DOCA was discovered, as the administration of DOCA not only preserves life but also allows the patient to lead a useful and active life. It was therefore decided to try liquorice in patients with Addison's disease – with most gratifying results.

The next step was to link the action of liquorice with that of cortisone which, incidentally, has largely replaced DOCA in the treatment of Addison's disease. This in turn led to the discovery that, not only had liquorice the same action as cortisone in retaining water in the body, and thereby causing oedema, but it also had another feature in common: what is known as an anti-inflammatory action. This is the basis for the use, not so much of cortisone, as of cortisone-like substances, of which there are now quite a number available: in the treatment, for example, of certain skin conditions and of certain conditions affecting the eye.

Here – before passing on to the final stage of the liquorice saga – would seem to be the place to draw attention to how all these modern discoveries about liquorice are confirming the uses to which it was put in the past. Its anti-inflammatory action explains why it earned its reputation for healing wounds, eye conditions, and the like. Even more interesting is the connection between this modern scientific evidence and the story of Theophrastus that by taking liquorice the Scythians were able to go for long periods without drinking. One explanation at least is that this was achieved as a result of liquorice causing retention of water in the body. If excretion of water in the urine was reduced as a result, then thirst would not arise, and there would be much less need to drink. Thus does legend become fact, and the twentieth century successor of the alchemist of old produce evidence to support the folklore of the great days of ancient Greece.

Finally, in this historical retrospect comes the modern evidence that liquorice has an anti-spasmodic action on the muscles of the stomach and bowel. Should this be the case, and the evidence is quite impressive, then we have an explanation of the age-old claim that it is of value in the alleviation of the pains of indigestion.

This last attribute, however, is not the explanation of the quite dramatic effect of liquorice in the treatment of gastric ulcer. This has been tracked down to a substance which has been synthesized from glycyrrhizin, and to which the name of carbenoxolone has been given. This, in the somewhat esoteric language (some would say jargon) of modern science, has been described as 'a pure synthetic derivative of one particular stereoisomer of a naturally occurring plant material – the product of natural synthesis suitably modified by chemical purification and derivatization'. In other words, it is what results when the scientist comes down off his hobby horse and devotes his attention to studying what Nature produces in the way of herbs that heal. A little more of this, and a little less dependence on synthesis *de novo*, would go far towards more and more efficient remedies for the ailments to which mankind is heir.

It is the same biochemists who go on to declare that 'carbenoxolone is a unique therapeutic entity, with equally remarkable properties in its biochemistry and molecular pharmacology'. Its claim to be 'a unique therapeutic entity' is, of course, its ability to accelerate the healing of gastric ulcers, an attribute possessed by no other known drug. One of its interesting features is that it is only effective in this way when taken by mouth. When given by injection it has an anti-inflammatory action equivalent to about one-third of the cortisone-like substance known as hydrocortisone, but no effect on a gastric ulcer. Conversely, when taken by mouth it has no anti-inflammatory action, but heals gastric ulcers. How it achieves this is still not quite clear, but it seems to be definitely a local action by the drug coming into direct contact with the ulcer.

This explains why hitherto it has proved relatively disappointing in the treatment of duodenal ulcers: that is, ulcers in the part of the gut immediately following the stomach. Carbenoxolone is rapidly absorbed into the body from the stomach, and there is none left to pass into the duodenum and exert its healing role there. To overcome this snag, an ingenious scheme has been evolved, whereby the drug is given in what is described as a 'position released' gelatin capsule. This is a capsule that swells in the stomach but does not rupture until after a period of two and a half to three hours, by which time it is in the part of the stomach known as the pyloric antrum, which is the part leading into the duodenum. There it finally bursts open and pours its contents of carbenoxolone straight into the duodenum where it is thus able to perform its healing action. That this is a true bill is indicated by an investigation in which the capsules were filled with radio-opaque material and given to volunteers. They were then studied by x-rays and the course of the capsules watched and photographed. In all eleven volunteers the capsules were seen to behave exactly as they were supposed to do; they swelled in the stomach without bursting until they arrived in the pyloric antrum when they ruptured two and a half to three hours after being swallowed and emptied themselves into the duodenum.

How effective it will prove in duodenal ulcers is still not quite clear, but in the case of gastric ulcers there is no doubt about its efficacy. As one expert has expressed it: 'Carbenoxolone facilitates the normal healing process, speeds it up and enables ulcers to heal in ambulatory patients at the same rate they would achieve if the patient stayed in bed. This', he notes, 'is of course a very considerable economic advantage.' As there are only two other known methods of accelerating the healing of gastric ulcers – rest in bed and cessation of smoking – this is no mean achievement. The only price to be paid for it is that carbenoxolone can produce the same side-effects as liquorice. It must therefore only be used under medical supervision. All the available evidence indicates, however, that used in this way there is seldom any difficulty in evolving a healing dose that has no side-effects.

Thus ends the liquorice story: yet another example of a herb that heals. From the Scythian sweet to carbenoxolone; from the liquorice all-sorts of our childhood to the drug that heals the ulcerated stomach; from the herb root used to flavour beer to the product of the modern pharmaceutical industry – these are all transitions that witness to the harvest that must still be awaiting the searching mind in this field of medicine.

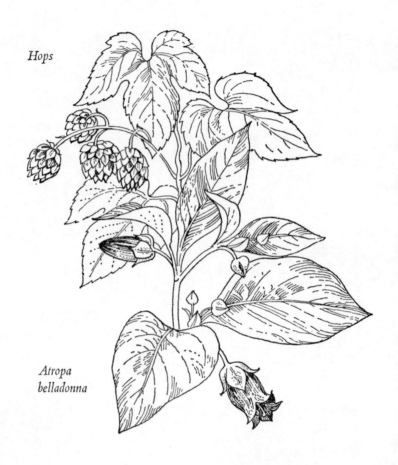

Hops

Atropa
belladonna

5

Herbs that soothe

Under the heading of 'Flower used as an anaesthetic', *The Times*, 10 October 1974, carried the following message, dated 9 October, from Hong Kong:

'China is successfully using an extract from the datura flower, a poisonous plant, for anaesthetizing the whole body during surgery, the New China News Agency said tonight.

The datura flower (thorn apple) is a member of the potato family.'

If a Chinese Rip Van Winkle had surfaced on 9 October 1974, after a sleep of a hundred times the duration of that of his American opposite number, he would have rubbed his eyes, not because things had changed so much since he had embarked on his long sleep, but because his fellow-countrymen were still using the same form of anaesthesia as when he went to sleep. What he probably would not have appreciated is that *Datura stramonium*, to give thorn apple its technical name, belongs to the botanical family, *Solanaceae*, which comprises eighty-five genera and around 2,300 species. Not only is the potato (*Solanum tuberosum*) one of these species, but so also are the tomato (*Solanum lycopersicum*) and tobacco (*Nicotiana tabacum*) as well as several of the many herbs that from very early times have soothed suffering pain-racked mankind to sleep and allowed many a surgical operation to be carried out under relatively painless conditions – if not the *de luxe* blissful oblivion the anaesthetics of today can induce in us before the surgeon's knife pierces our skin. Among these herbs that soothe are the deadly nightshade (*Atropa belladonna*) and henbane (*Hyoscyamus niger*).

That our forebears should have been such ardent searchers after herbs that relieve, or at least ease, pain is not surprising. Pain has always been with us from the beginning of time, and it is one thing we share with the entire range of Nature, plants and herbs included. Much though we may loathe, hate and detest it, however, it is one of the essentials of life. If there were no pain, there would be no life. It is Nature's warning that there is something wrong – the red light that warns us to take evading action : whether this be the simple reflex of quickly withdrawing our hand from something that is burning it, removing the thorn we have picked up in our foot, or calling in the doctor because of the unbearable pain in our abdomen which turns out to be acute appendicitis, which, if not operated on, may well prove fatal.

The classical, and all too topical, example today is the heart pain we know as angina pectoris. This can be one of the most agonizing, and at times terrifying, pains to which man is heir; yet it is fundamentally beneficial. It is a warning from our heart that we are overdoing it. If we obey the warning and rest, the pain immediately begins to fade away and, if in the future we restrict the amount of exercise we take, then the pain will not recur and we know that we are keeping within the capacity of the heart. On the other hand, if we ignore the warning the overstrained heart finally gives up the hopeless struggle, with a resulting coronary thrombosis – or even sudden death.

Useful – indeed essential – warning though it be, there are occasions when it must be brought under control once its cause has been detected, and is being dealt with if humanly possible, whether by operation as in the case of injury or cancer, or by medical treatment as in the case of colic due to stones in the kidney. In other words, the essential rule for the treatment of pain is find and remove the cause. While this is being achieved, or where the cause cannot be found or is irremovable, then treat the pain.

For such alleviation, as man, like animals, early discovered, the fundamental rule is rest. The wounded animal retires to his den to lick his wounds and rest them, knowing that this is the surest and quickest way of obtaining relief. Man, however, was not satisfied with this simple procedure. He had a mind that resented pain much more than the animals, and he was determined to do everything possible to speed up the alleviation of the underlying cause or to obtain relief by other methods. Having no precedents, and having to learn everything *de novo*, the process was a slow one of evolution by trial and error, probably starting off with the observation that exposure of an injured limb to the cold water of lake or river brought relief. Later, or simultaneously, the soothing effect of heat was probably realized as a result of exposure of the injured painful part to the sun and, once the soothing effect of heat was appreciated, then would follow the use of heat from fires and stoves for this purpose. And so, as he moved up the scale of progress and his imagination developed, there evolved demons responsible for pain of unknown cause and medicine men and priests and finally there came Christianity with its sublimation of these primeval instincts into divine healing through touch and prayer, or prayer alone.

But ancient man, and probably primitive man as well, was not satisfied with what we would now call physiotherapy and faith healing. As soon as he realized that herbs could help to make life more bearable by easing his indigestion, his cough and the inflammation of his eyes, he turned to them for relief of his pain. His search was not in vain. How many mistakes he made we know not; neither is it recorded how many deaths or near-deaths resulted from his experimentation. Records did not exist in those days; neither were there those interfering Medical Commissions to cramp his style. Yet, whether by fair means or foul, by accident or good luck, by careful observation or shrewd deducation, in due course he had collected a useful pain-relieving pharma-copoeia, including, among many others, the poppy, henbane, hemp, and mandragora.

Probably one of the earliest written records is that on a Baby-lonian clay tablet of around 2250 BC, recommending a cement of powdered henbane seeds and gum mastic as a filling of a dental cavity for the relief of toothache. A later development was that of the ancient Scythians who breathed the fumes produced by heated *Cannabis indica* to induce a state of mental exaltation, not the least important attribute of which was that it rendered them oblivious to all but the most racking pain. By the time of the Christian era the use of pain-relieving herbs was much more widespread. According to the Gospels the 'potion of the con-demned', traditionally offered to the victims of crucifixion to help relieve their agonies and which Christ refused on the Cross, consisted of either wine or vinegar mingled with gall, myrrh or hyssop, though it is of more than passing interest that, while Matthew, Mark and John all refer to the constituents, Luke, the physician, is silent on this point. Is this an early example of pro-fessional reticence such as would appeal to the disciplinary dons of the General Medical Council?

Before reviewing some of these traditional pain-relieving herbs, it is meet that some attention should be given to a much misunderstood subject: that of surgical anaesthesia. The popular belief which is shared by some of our more cynical medical historians, is that this only dates back a hundred years or so to the introduction of ether as an anaesthetic in the USA in 1846. This is certainly the case so far as modern anaesthesia is concerned; but not all of those who dogmatize on this point are aware that ether was described as long ago as 1540 – that is, three centuries before it surfaced again in the USA – and that, according to Professor Chauncey D Leake, no mean medical historian, 'there is indication that its "sleep-producing" properties were known about the time of its discovery'.

This rules out, or certainly argues against, the thesis that has been advanced by some, that up until a century or so ago our forebears were more interested in the infliction than the relief of pain, and that they accepted pain as a matter of course. Should that be the case, then it is difficult to understand why so much legend and allegory, from the *Odyssey* onwards, should dwell on pain-relieving and sleep-inducing herbs as in, for example, the tale of Helen, the daughter of Zeus, when she prepares a potion to forget pain and grief in the oblivion of sleep. More probable is it that many of the unauthenticated horror tales of operations carried out by brute force without any attempt to reduce pain are grossly exaggerated. No-one will deny that the butchery of army surgery in the Middle Ages must have been hell on earth for the unfortunate soldiery, but all the evidence suggests that mankind has always been searching for some means of making surgery as painless as possible.

Professor Chauncey Leake, for instance, recounts how the early Inca shamans, or medicine-men, dating from around AD 1000 used the pain-relieving properties of coca leaves (the source of cocaine, still one of our best local anaesthetics) in trephining skulls. This they did by chewing the leaves and allowing their saliva to drop in the area of the skull to be operated on. Crude, possibly, by modern standards, but ingenious. Incidentally, it is worthy of note, as evidence of the extent to which the medical study of herbs had been developed in South America at this period, that when the Spaniards conquered the land they found lists of over 3,000 plants used by the Aztecs in the treatment of disease.

But the tradition of anaesthesia for the relief of pain in operations goes back to the early days of most of the ancient civilizations – Greek, Roman, Hindu and Chinese. Whether Greek god or man of Epidaurus, Aesculapius is attributed with using a potion known as nepenthe to produce insensibility in those operated on, and Dioscorides, the Greek physician of the first century AD, who served as a surgeon with Nero's army, refers in his *Materia Medica* to the use of mandragora wine for those 'upon whom they wish to produce anaesthesia while being cut or cauterized'. The ancient Hindus, too, used concoctions of pain-relieving herbs to ease the pain of patients about to undergo surgery, as did the ancient Chinese. Thus, of Hua T'a, who was born around AD 200, and described by Professor Ralph H Major, the distinguished American medical historian, as 'the most famous surgeon in Chinese history', Professor Major says that 'his fame rests chiefly upon his employment of anaesthetics and upon his great surgical skill'. The composition of his anaesthetic, which was given by mouth, is not known, but it has been suggested that it may have been *Cannabis indica*. To quote Professor Major again, 'Chinese physicians employed for this purpose *Datura alba*, *Rhododendron sinense*, *Jasmine sambac* and *Aconite.*'

The first reference to the use of herbs to induce anaesthesia in Britain seems to date from the twelfth century, when there is a reference to a preparation of unknown constitution, known as letarigon, being used for those 'who suffered incision and sometimes burning [cauterization] of the limbs and the abrasion even of the vitals, and after wakening from the sleep have been ignorant of what was done to them'. The following century an English Franciscan, Bartolomeus Anglicus, suggested that mandrake in

74

wine could deaden sensation during an operation. Another physician of the thirteenth century, Gilbertus Anglicus, recommended a method he had learned at Salerno, then the great medical school of Europe. This was the use of a so-called soporific sponge which, in the *Antidotarium* of Nicolas of Salerno, written in the twelfth century, is described as follows:

'Take ... of opium, thebaicum, juice of hyoscyamine, unripened berry of the blackberry, lettuce seed, juice of hemlock, poppy, mandragora, ivy ... Put these all together in a vessel and plunge therein a new sea-sponge just as it comes from the sea, taking care that fresh water does not touch it. And put this in the sun during the dog-days until all the liquid is consumed. And when there is need, dip it a little in water not too warm, and apply it to the nostrils of the patient, and he will quickly go to sleep. When, moreover, you want to awaken him, apply juice from the root of the fennel and he will soon bestir himself.'

There were variations in the herbs used in these soporific sponges and, while they were obviously used primarily to induce sleep, there seems little doubt that they were also used to induce anaesthesia as we know it. The obvious snag about them, of course, is whether any of the active constituents were volatile enough to be inhaled, but some may have been swallowed if the sponge was held over the mouth as well as the nose. There may also have been an element of what is known as carbon dioxide narcosis brought about by the patient not being able to breathe on account of the nose and mouth being covered, thereby resulting in an accumulation of carbon dioxide in the blood, which is known to produce anaesthesia. Whatever the rationale or the efficiency of the method, however, there would appear to be little doubt that surgical anaesthesia was practised long before the days of ether and chloroform, using a wide variety of pain-relieving herbs. Whether or not anything like adequate anaesthesia was induced, there can be no doubt about the efficiency of many of these herbs as relievers of pain.

Of the opium poppy (*Papaver somniferum*) nothing can be said that is not already known. It is the oldest and still the best reliever of pain, which man, with all his ingenuity, has not been able to improve on, and it is one of the few essential drugs in the *Pharmacopoeia*. Why Nature should have given it such a dreadful converse to its brilliant soothing properties is one of those unsolved mysteries of life. Is it part of the penalty that mankind has to pay for his breaking the fundamental rules of life? Be all that as it philosophically may, there is no doubt of the devastation it can cause when abused. There are, however, some in the medical profession who wonder whether the pendulum has not swung too far in the way of penalizing that great part of the population who would benefit from its use when indicated but are deprived of it because of the over-concern of the do-gooders in and out of Parliament with that small minority of the populace whose instability of character converts them so easily into drug addicts.

Almost equally old is mandrake, or mandragora, a native of Syria, which for long enjoyed a reputation as a reliever of pain. Shakespeare's 'drowsy syrup' and a regular inhabitant of the medieval monastery herb gardens, it is scarcely ever used today, although recent investigations indicate that it contains several of the solanaceous alkaloids, which would well explain its claim to a niche in the temple of nepenthe.

The *Solanaceae*, as already indicated, is a botanical family which includes some of the best known, and most notorious, herbs in the whole history of medicine. They include atropine, or belladonna, henbane, hyoscyamus, hyoscine, and stramonium, or thorn apple, as well as mandrake. All possess sedative properties by virtue of a depressing action on the brain, but some of them are liable to go to the opposite extreme and produce delirium and hallucinations. Hence their dreaded reputation in the Middle Ages as constituents of the witches' brews which so intrigued and terrified our forebears. Some of them, such as thorn apple, are traditional hallucenogenic agents among the Indians of Central and South America. In spite of much active investigation, which has isolated some of the more active and useful constituents such as hyoscine, still the best travel sickness remedy, and, with morphine, the producer of the 'twilight sleep' so beloved of the fashionable mothers of the 'tween-war era, who preferred their own comfort during parturition to the welfare of their resultingly drugged offspring, there is still obviously much scope for research into the constitution of some of the herbs in this heterogeneous collection and their effect on the mind.

Two other pain-relieving drugs have come down to us from the past. One, aconite, monkshood or wolfsbane (a name derived from the fact that in the Middle Ages it was used as a poison bait for wolves), was rightly eschewed by the herbalists of old who described it as 'the queen mother of poisons', a phrase which *Martindale* translates into modern terminology as 'a dangerous therapeutic agent'. It does, however, have a sedative and narcotic action, and two species, including that known as yellow wolfsbane, are used in China as a narcotic and sedative.

The other consists of several species of *Ipomoea*, a curiously mixed genus which includes jalap, one of the drastic purgatives used as an antidote by our over-eating and over-drinking Victorian forebears. The species of interest here are those known as morning glory. One of these (*Ipomoea violacea*) came to us from South America where, as ololiuqui, the natives have for long used it for its hallucenogenic properties. Another, bush morning glory (*Ipomoea leptophylla*), which grows on the western side of the North American continent, is traditionally used by the local Indians who burn the roots and inhale the smoke as a remedy for nervousness and nightmares, just as a traditional domestic remedy in Europe for toothache is to throw seeds of henbane (*Hyoscyamus niger*) on hot coal and inhale the vapour through the mouth. It may well be that a more intensive study of these two sets of herbs might produce some as yet unknown sedative or pain-relieving drug.

A safer soother, and one used widely until quite recently, is gelsemium or yellow jasmine root, a plant indigenous to the southern USA, chiefly Virginia, the Carolinas and Tennessee. It is not to be confused with *Jasminum nudiflorum*, the yellow-flowering jasmine cultivated in Britain, though one species of jasmine (*Jasminum lanceolatum*) is used as an analgesic, or pain reliever, in China. Gelsemium, usually in a mixture named Gowers' mixture after Sir William Gowers, the great British neurologist who first introduced it, was for a long time the traditional prescription for trigeminal neuralgia and migraine. It may have been replaced by more effective drugs for these two conditions, but it is still a useful sedative contribution from the world of herbs.

On a slightly less orthodox level come two plants which no longer receive the official approbation of the orthodox medical profession. One is chamomile, an old domestic remedy which only disappeared from the *British Pharmaceutical Codex* some twenty years ago. It has a double claim to fame: making lawns as well as making useful medicines. It is claimed, apparently with a considerable degree of evidence, that the lawn on which Drake played his famous game of bowls was a chamomile lawn, and chamomile lawns are still to be found in Royal parks as well as in the garden of Buckingham Palace. This use of chamomile lawns dates back to Elizabethan days, the basis of their popularity being that they were easy to establish and maintain, resisted dry spells, and gave off a scent reminiscent of apples; hence the name which comes from two Greek words meaning 'apple on the ground'.

Medicinally its more traditional use was as a soothing sedative tea, though it was also claimed that bathing any part of the body that 'was weary and in pain' in chamomile brought welcome relief. The reputation of chamomile tea survived longer in Europe than in Britain; today the Italians, who apparently drink a million cups of it a day, have converted it into big business, demanding the cultivation of vast acreages in Italy, Hungary, Poland, Rumania, Bulgaria, Egypt and the Argentine. To such an extent has this demand for chamomile grown that one Italian company recently reported having an annual turnover of over £3 million from its sale. Today, apparently, the ladies of Italy drink it to ease stomach troubles, while their menfolk drink it in bars in the evening as an insurance against insomnia, and the elderly like it as a nightcap with a mildly soporific effect. An enterprising Italian company, sensing the commercial possibilities of this reputation, are now marketing it under the slogan of 'cup of serenity' with the claim that it is:

'One of nature's mildest and most effective sedatives and tranquillizers, available at only a fraction of the price of the pharmaceutical drugs which humans are swallowing in enormous and growing volume to calm their collective nerves.'

Is this the opportunity for family doctors – especially those in country areas – to switch over from expensive tranquillizers to the old-fashioned chamomile tea for their patients, to whom a 'cup of serenity' would be a welcome boon? Or perhaps the local pharmacist might try this as a sideline to help in keeping down the nation's drug bill.

To the modern generation the lettuce is merely a standard British vegetable greenery for a salad, but our predecessors had much more respect for it as a soother of pain and an inducer of sleep when opium was either not available or was considered inadvisable. This opiate-like action was obtained in several ways. The simplest, widely practised at one time, was for those troubled with insomnia to eat a lettuce the last thing at night. Alternatively,

79

a common country practice was to drink a cup of lettuce tea on going to bed. A more scientific approach was based on the fact that the common lettuce (*Lactuca virosa*) contains a white bitter latex which exudes from the plant when it is wounded. This latex, when dried, is named lettuce-opium (or *lactucarium*). It is light green in colour when fresh, later turning brown when it gives off a characteristic opium-like odour. Incorporated in pastilles or lozenges, it is used as a sedative for irritating or hacking coughs.

Yet another example of its use was recorded recently in *The Times*, when a correspondent wrote that her great-great-grandfather, Dr James Murdoch, practised medicine in Van Diemen's Land from 1822 to 1848. According to a family memoir, when supplies of opium were not available, 'he sent to the garden for some lettuces, crushed them in a pestle, and extracted an opiate from them'. As the correspondent nicely adds: 'Did not Beatrix Potter in *The Tale of The Flopsy Bunnies* remark on the "soporific effect of eating too much lettuce"?'

This review of some of the many herbs that soothe began with the poppy, the most potent of them all. It is appropriate therefore that it should end with another which shares its disturbing addictive properties, and with the one which led to the discovery of the most widespread of all the so-called analgesics. The addiction-forming drug is cocaine, which consists of the dried leaves of *Erythroxylum coca* (Bolivian or Huanuco leaf) or *E. truxillense* (Peruvian or Truxillo leaf). These are the famous coca leaves which the natives of South America, since the days of the Incas (though originally they were reserved for their chiefs) have chewed to give them the staying power to perform their arduous tasks, by allaying the pangs of hunger and the feeling of fatigue. In those early days, too, as noted earlier in this chapter, its anaesthetic properties were appreciated; but although it was introduced to Europe in 1688, the active constituent was not isolated until

1859. Yet another quarter of a century was to pass before Dr Carl Koller, of Vienna, finally put it on the anaesthetic map as what the *British Pharmaceutical Codex* now describes as 'the oldest local anaesthetic'. Other better and safer ones may have been introduced but, in spite of its addiction proclivities, cocaine still holds its place.

And so to that most widely used of all domestic remedies for the relief of aches and pains, no matter where they may be – namely aspirin. This synthetic drug – acetylsalicylic acid, to give it its chemical name – which first appeared in 1899, we owe to the age-old reputation of the bark of various species of willow trees for easing 'the ague'. These trees flourish all over the world, and wherever they are found the locals have discovered their efficacy, and particularly that of the bark, for relieving the aches and pains of mankind, particularly those at one time known as the ague, and now as the rheumatics.

The modern history of aspirin dates back to 1763 when there appeared in the *Philosophical Transactions of the Royal Society of London* a communication from the Rev. Edward Stone of Chipping Norton, Oxfordshire – one of those country divines who used to combine so effectively the care of the soul with that of the body, as well as with the study of science. In this he extolled 'the wonderful efficacy of this Cortex Salignus [willow bark] in agues and intermitting cases'. His reasons for first investigating the efficacy of willow bark were twofold. In the first place its bitter taste was reminiscent of that of Peruvian bark, the source of what we now know as quinine, which was already known in those days to be an effective treatment of what is now called malaria. In the second place, to use his own pleasing language:

'As the tree delights in a moist or wet soil, where agues chiefly abound, the general maxim, that many natural remedies carry their cures along with them, or that their remedies lie

81

not far from their causes, was so very appropriate to this
particular case, that I could not help applying it.'

Wrong though his premises may have been, his logic led to the
right answer, and the derivatives of the bark of the willow tree
were launched on a career that was to end just over one hundred
years later in the discovery of aspirin – not as a remedy for
malaria (for many years the prerogative of quinine) but as the
prince of alleviators of those rheumatic pains that dog the life of
mankind throughout his earthly career.

The first definitive step in this progression came early in the
nineteenth century, when one of the first achievements of modern
chemistry in the drug field was the isolation from willow bark
of its active principle, to which the name of salicin was given.
From this, in due course, was isolated salicylic acid which was
finally synthesized in 1852. Then things began to move at an ever-
increasing pace, and by the end of the century both salicylic acid
and salicin had been shown to be most effective drugs in the treatment of various rheumatic conditions, particularly rheumatic
fever, then one of the great scourges of childhood as the cause of a
steady stream of children with crippled hearts.

Unfortunately, salicylic acid and salicin had a most unpleasantly
bitter taste, almost impossible to disguise, and also a marked
tendency to irritate the stomach. German chemists therefore got
busy in an attempt to produce a derivative which would be as
effective but less upsetting. This they finally did in 1899 in the
form of acetylsalicylic acid, to which the company gave the trade
name of aspirin. People often wonder how trade names are
produced. So do doctors. As often as not there is no rhyme or
reason about the process except that it is either a catching name or
refers to the action of the preparation. In this respect, aspirin can
claim a somewhat more scientific, some would say typically
Teutonic, origin. The prefix, 'a', stands for the acetyl in the name;

the root, 'spir', stands for spirsaüme, the German for salicylic acid, while the suffix, 'in', rounds off the word.

During the next half-century it climbed rapidly to the top of the medical popularity poll as a pain reliever, or analgesic, for all types of rheumatic pain, of serious diseases such as rheumatic fever and rheumatoid arthritis, of what the laity describe as their rheumatics, of gout, and of the ubiquitous headache to which modern mankind is so prone. As one writer has put it: 'As an analgesic it relieves pain rapidly, inexpensively and effectively.'

During this half-century, in spite of its widespread use, and in spite of much intensive research, no evidence could be found as to how it worked. Then quite suddenly the problem was solved by the discovery of a hitherto unknown group of substances, to which the name of prostaglandins was given. These, it was found, were responsible for producing fever and those painful inflammatory changes in the tissues of the body which, amongst other things, are responsible for what we know as rheumatic pains. In other words, they produce the very things relieved by aspirin. Was it possible, the research workers asked, that aspirin relieved pain, inflammation and fever by preventing, or at least reducing, the production of prostaglandins? The answer was in the affirmative, and the age-old mystery of the *modus operandi* of the bark of the willow tree, and its modern successor, was solved.

But this was by no means the end of the road. Rather was it the beginning of a new era in the history of aspirin, and for the simple reason that it was found that these prostaglandins affected the working of the body in many ways, including, for example, stimulating the uterus, or womb, to contract. For this reason it is now used to induce abortions. If prostaglandins act in this way, is it possible that they may be responsible for inducing unwanted abortions or miscarriages? If so, is it possible that aspirin might be able to prevent such miscarriages and abortions?

This is a point still to be decided, but there is a growing volume of evidence of the possible value of aspirin in preventing clotting of the blood, and in this way it may be of value in preventing those heart attacks that have become such a scourge of western civilization. Preliminary trials in Cardiff, Boston and Frankfurt suggest, though they do not prove, that this may well be the case, and the Royal College of General Practitioners has embarked on a national investigation to decide whether or not this is a true bill. Equally intriguing is the possibility, now being investigated at the Royal Marsden Hospital, London, that aspirin may be of some value in the prevention, and treatment, of certain forms of cancer. In the words of the director of the research team carrying out this work, 'It is early days, but the results are encouraging.'

What western civilization would do without aspirin (it is reckoned that 5,000 to 6,000 million tablets are consumed every year in Britain alone: enough to provide each person with 100 tablets a year) it is difficult to imagine, and with these exciting new discoveries, it is almost taking on the attributes of what the so-called communications media love to call a 'wonder drug'. It may not be a herb, but it is doubtful whether mankind would have thought out the formula on its own, and therefore to the willow tree must go the credit for all that aspirin does to soothe the aches and pains of suffering humanity, many of which are induced by the excesses to which we allow modern life to drive us on too many occasions.

But perhaps the very last word should go to what to many must appeal as the most soothing of all remedies – herb pillows. It seems such a natural, if irrational, use, and it is one that has stood the test of time. Hops can probably claim the widest use in this sleep-inducing practice. The secret of success lies in not packing the pillow, or the bag of soft muslin which is secured to the pillow by tacking threads, too tightly, so that, as one expert has put it, 'the fragrant pillow yields deliciously to the ear'. The dried hops have to be renewed every four to six weeks. Perhaps the most distinguished patient submitted to this form of sedation was George III during his relapses into mental instability. The concept of hops as sedatives was strongly backed up by the Cockney hop pickers who remained convinced that the powerful odour of the hop gardens lulled their infants to sleep.

One of the claims made for hop pillows is that they induce 'sound and natural sleep'. And what more could one ask for even if, as the cynics contend, the *modus operandi* is suggestion? Sleep is none the less sound and refreshing because it is produced by suggestion. Indeed, in this barbiturate- and tranquillizer-ridden age it might well be claimed that sleep induced by harmless suggestion is more physiological than that induced by the potentially dangerous synthetic products of today. Hops are not the only contents of herbal pillows. Other herbs that have been recommended are lady's mantle (*Alchemilla vulgaris*), mint, and sweet woodruff which is also used in the Netherlands to stuff mattresses. On occasions a combination of herbs was recommended, as in the following eighteenth century recipe:

> 'Take of cowslips and fresh hops, newly dried, as many as you deem enough to make a soft stuffed cushion in equal parts. Distribute your hops and cowslips nicely in a bowl and proceed to stuff your pillow until you feel it comfortable to the head.'

Suggestion it may be (like the advice the wise old nanny gave to her charge who wanted to have sweet dreams: 'Go to sleep with a smile on your face'), but a pleasing thought in these days of arid materialism and feckless chasing after hallucinogenic wills-o'-the-wisp.

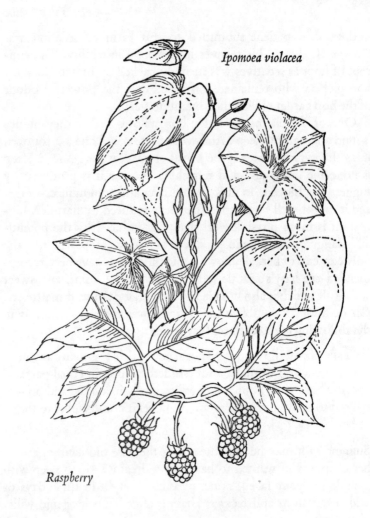

Ipomoea violacea

Raspberry

6
The ergot epic

Moulds and fungi may be the bane of our lives, with their proclivity for flourishing at the expense of objects which we treasure or food which we can often ill-afford to lose. As the searching mind of medicine, however, has probed ever deeper into the mysteries of Nature, it has revealed that these humble, and hitherto spurned, products can be among the most valuable servants of mankind. Penicillin, of course, is the classical example, but even more fascinating is ergot. Strictly speaking it is not a herb, but it is so closely integrated with the plant world that it always has been dealt with in this connection. Hence its inclusion among the herbs that heal.

With a long, and initially unpleasantly dishonourable, history, it has in the end proved to be a veritable treasure box – although at times it has threatened to turn out a Pandora's box – of potent and valuable drugs. To date, some two dozen alkaloids have been isolated from it. From the therapeutic point of view, these can be divided into three main broad categories: those used in midwifery; those used in the relief of migraine; and those with a hallucinogenic action. A more variegated spectrum of therapeutic activity it would be difficult to imagine, but it is a salutary reminder that the human body must be regarded as a whole, and not merely as a collation of isolated parts, such as a brain, a heart, a liver, and so forth. As a corollary it should make us chary of automatically rejecting, as the sceptics so often do, the claims of folklore medicine on the grounds that it makes out so many merits for an individual herb. Granted that these claims are often absurdly wild, and that 'heal-alls' – a favourite description in medieval times – are few and far between, but a herb (or drug) with a single isolated action is almost as rare. All this, however, does not detract from the intriguing versatility of the products of ergot but, before reviewing them in the classification given, its history and fundamental characteristics call for attention.

Ergot is the hard, resistant, resting stage, or sclerotium, of the fungus, *Claviceps purpurea*, which parasitizes rye. It can grow on other grasses as well, but the ergot used in medicine is that obtained from rye. Careful husbandry has so reduced the incidence of this fungus infestation that crops artificially infected with the fungus have now to be cultivated; a method of semi-synthesis is also now available.

At one time, however, the fungus was rampant and widespread and, as rye was the predominant cereal in Europe, the results were often catastrophic, resulting in what has been described as the 'infamous' history of ergot. This dates back to as early as 600 BC, an Assyrian tablet from that period alluding to a 'noxious pustule in the ear of grain'.

It was in the Middle Ages, however, that ergot had its heyday, causing recurrent epidemics of what is now known as ergotism, but was then known as St Anthony's fire, *ignis sacer* (holy fire) or *mal des ardents*, resulting from eating rye contaminated by the ergot fungus. The disease took two forms, which, curiously enough, rarely occurred together. The most common was characterized by agonizing pain in the extremities (hence the names, sacred fire and the like) leading on to gangrene of the affected limbs. The other, and rarer, type gave rise to paroxysmal epileptic-like convulsions.

So widespread was the condition in the south of France that in 1093 a religious Order was instituted for the purpose of caring for the victims of the disease, and the Order chose St Anthony as its patron saint: hence the name given to the disease of St Anthony's fire. Some idea of the extent of the outbreaks can be obtained from the fact that in the south of France alone in 994 there were 40,000 deaths, while 1200 died in an outbreak in Cambrai in 1129. There were also three major outbreaks in Germany in the sixteenth century, but after the recognition of the cause in the following century, the incidence fell, and only minor sporadic outbreaks occurred, though these have continued until quite recent times. The interesting suggestion has recently been made that the famous Salem witchcraft trials in Massachusetts in 1692 may have been the result of an outbreak of ergotism. The disease was never common in Britain, presumably because little rye is grown on this side of the English Channel.

Even while these dreaded outbreaks of ergotism were occurring, we find the original reference to the use of ergot in midwifery – the sphere in which it was first to achieve recognition as a valuable drug rather than a dangerous contaminant. Towards the end of the sixteenth century a German physician referred to the fact that ergot was being used by midwives for quickening labour. Thus began a story which redounds to the credit of the family doctor, and illustrates well how the pharmaceutical industry, backed up, let it in all fairness be added, by the academic backroom boys in their ivory towers, can be so badly off beam. It is the story of how ergot came to play a valuable role in the quickening of labour pains and the control and prevention of that dreaded complication of labour – haemorrhage after the birth of the child, or post-partum haemorrhage as it is known.

Although the use of ergot for this purpose dates back to the sixteenth century, what might be described as the modern era began in 1808, when Dr John Stearns of New York published a report entitled *An Account of the Pulvis Parturiens*. The active agent in this powder was ergot, and Dr Stearns recommended it for the quickening of labour. In 1824, another American, Dr Hosack, recommended caution in its use, and advised that this should be restricted to the control of post-partum haemorrhage. In this capacity it soon caught on, and for the next century there can have been few parturient ladies who did not end their confinement with a dose of liquid extract of ergot – and with most satisfying results.

In due course, needless to say, the pharmaceutical industry stepped in, and got their chemists and pharmacologists on the job. The first result of this came in 1906, when two research workers of a British pharmaceutical company reported the isolation from ergot of an active alkaloid, which they named ergotoxine. Twelve years later a Swiss pharmaceutical company surfaced with another active alkaloid, christened ergotamine. In due course the two turned out to have identical properties, but the two companies differed violently – and in public – on their relative clinical properties.

Here the Swiss company had the strong practical advantage that British obstetricians had cold-shouldered ergotoxine, whereas the Swiss company, with that national genius that has brought so much financial success to the four Swiss pharmaceutical giants, obtained maximum co-operation for clinical trials in Germany, Switzerland and elsewhere, and in relatively little time ergotamine was selling like hot cakes. The British company, though cold-shouldered, was not to be outdone, and a 'handbook' was circulated to doctors, the gist of which was as follows:

'The characteristic pharmacological therapeutic action of ergot is due to the alkaloid ergotoxine. The specific physiological effect and therapeutic efficiency of any preparation of ergot depends on the presence of this active principle. Many preparations of ergot are highly unsatisfactory and some are without any therapeutic action whatever because they contain no ergotoxine.'

In view of subsequent events, no more blatant example of scientific falsehood could be imagined.

British obstetricians and midwives, however, refused to give up their *British Pharmacopoeia* preparation, liquid extract of ergot, on which they had been born and bred professionally, and which had proved such a valuable adjunct to the successful culmination of parturition. Finally, the problem was handed over to Dr Chassar Moir (later Professor of Obstetrics in Oxford), then an obstetric registrar at University College Hospital, London, by the Therapeutic Trials Committee of the Medical Research Council. In due course, in a brilliant triad of reports published in the *British Medical Journal*, he showed:

(a)   In 1932, that ergotoxine and ergotamine were powerful stimulants of the uterus, causing it to contract when given by injection, but were relatively inactive when given by mouth.

(b)   In a second report in 1932, that the liquid extract of ergot, as prepared by the specification of the *British Pharmacopoeia*, had a potent action in stimulating the uterus to contract after labour was completed. He added: 'There is reason to believe that the characteristic and traditional effect of ergot is due to a substance as yet unidentified.'

(c)   In 1935, in a joint report with Dr H W Dudley, came the solution of the mystery, summarized in the authors' own words: 'We believed that the clinician was fully vindicated

in his dogged belief in the efficiency of the old fashioned preparation. In spite of some criticism and scepticism [a masterly
understatement] our clinical and chemical observations kept
us convinced of the truth of our conclusions, and we are now
able to prove their correctness by reporting the isolation of
the substance to which ergot rightly owes its long-estab-
lished reputation as the "pulvis parturiens". We propose to
name it "ergometrine".'

In other words, both the British and Swiss pharmaceutical companies were wrong. The alkaloid they had isolated had nothing
to do with the value of ergot in midwifery. This action was due
to the alkaloid isolated by Dr Chassar Moir and Dr Dudley,
which was present in the liquid extract of ergot, which the
British and Swiss companies had slanged, but which doctors and
midwives refused to give up.

So were the mighty academics and industrialists shattered, and
the 'dogged' clinician proved to be right. Would that this had
happened more often in the past, and that the clinician had been
prepared to stick to his own experience rather than be inveigled,
browbeaten, or bamboozled, as in the case of digitalis, for instance,
into accepting the facile tales of the academic pharmacologist
or the smooth medical 'rep'.

A somewhat similar story, but without such a happy ending,
is that of raspberry tea. Sir Beckwith Whitehouse, when Professor of Obstetrics in the University of Birmingham, had his
attention drawn to the fact that in certain areas of Herefordshire
and Worcestershire it was a common practice for women to use
an infusion of raspberry leaves to allay the pains of labour. The
same tea was also used, with apparently satisfactory results, in
severe cases of dysmenorrhoea, or painful menstruation.

He referred the problem to Professor J H Burn, the Professor
of Pharmacology at the University of Oxford. In the course of his

preliminary investigations Professor Burn found that raspberry-leaf tea had been a herbalist's remedy for many years and noted that 'it is said to be the best known and oldest of all the herb infusions and to be included as proved aid in maternity in the most ancient of herbal books'. That it still retained its reputation was evident from the statement from a firm of herb specialists which he quotes:

'The leaves give to the infusion an odour and flavour somewhat similar to that of some kinds of black tea. Raspberry leaves have astringent properties and also act as a stimulant. It is found that if the infusion be taken freely before and during confinement, parturition is easy and speedy.'

In due course Professor Burn found scientific experimental evidence to support these claims, in that a preparation of raspberry leaves had a definite action on the uterus of the cat, rabbit and guinea-pig, causing it to contract or relax. He suggested that there were probably two different principles concerned, one causing relaxation, and the other causing contraction, of the uterus, and he concluded that 'the principle causing relaxation is probably the basis of the traditional use of raspberry tea for making activity of the uterus less painful', and that this principle should be 'valuable in relieving painful menstruation due to spasmodic uterine contraction'.

On the basis of these pharmacological findings, Sir Beckwith Whitehouse tried it in patients, and in a report published in 1941 gave details of three women, in all of whom it diminished contractions of the uterus following childbirth. His conclusion was that in fragarine, as he had christened this active principle,

'we have available an active principle that may have a useful clinical application in the treatment of irregular uterine contraction during labour and menstruation'. He added: 'In the absence, as yet, of any more elegant preparation, crude raspberry-leaf tea is being used in one of the Worcestershire maternity hospitals, and the nursing staff report favourably upon its effect in "making things easier".'

I decided to take up this clue, and wrote to the present incumbent of the Birmingham Chair of Obstetrics. He wrote back to tell me that he 'had no information except that there were no converts among Sir Beckwith's colleagues here', but he also passed on my letter to Sir Beckwith's obstetrical son who replied:

'I remember well my father talking about fragarine in my early days as a medical student ... As I remember it, the development of ergometrine which took place about much the same time and was a far more effective drug over-shadowed fragarine, in which interest lapsed. I believe I am right in saying that raspberry-leaf tea is still used among the gipsies and Black Country people in the Worcestershire and Staffordshire area with a view to expediting labour.'

As I knew that Sir John Stallworthy, Professor Chassar Moir's successor as Nuffield Professor of Obstetrics in the University of Oxford, had also done some work on the subject, I wrote to him also, and received the following reply:

'Our work with raspberry-leaf tea was finally abandoned. By that time two active principles had been isolated, one of which appeared to stimulate uterine activity, and the other to bring about relaxation. No results were published, and I regret this, but we had really not progressed to the stage of solving the difficulties in purifying the preparations and making them safe for quantitative trials. I hope some day somebody will do this, because there seems to be sufficient folklore, and also veterinary experience, to suggest that raspberry leaf has properties which can make labour easier.'

So there the story ends, at least for the time being, intriguingly inviting some up and coming young obstetrician to take up the problem and decide whether or not the raspberry leaf deserves this obstetrical reputation, which is by no means confined to the Midlands and West Country. In his fascinating reminiscences, *Country Doctor*, Dr Geoffrey Barber, the doyen of Essex general practice, recalls: 'There was a popular superstition that "raspberry-leaf tea" would make labour easier, and young wives were encouraged by their mothers to drink it regularly as their time got nearer; if all went well, the tea and grandma were given the credit.' Neither is the pharmacological evidence confined to Oxford. Investigators at Chelsea College (London University) have reported comparable findings.

Here then is another example of a herb that heals. Its final acceptance into orthodox practice still awaits further evidence, but it is clear that the old wives' tales about its value have at least a modicum of justification. Surely in these days, when meddlesome midwifery (anathema to the older generation of obstetricians) is becoming increasingly prevalent, there is more than an urgent need to investigate the merits, or demerits, of an old-established and apparently safe, practice such as this. Such investigations might well yield us a safe and useful addition to our therapeutic armamentarium.

While midwifery is the traditional field in which ergot achieved fame, as already indicated it acts on many other parts of the body in addition to the uterus. It is two of these further modes of action that are used in the treatment of migraine: its ability to constrict blood vessels and its action antagonistic to a substance which plays an important part in the metabolism and working of the brain – serotonin. Although the precise cause of migraine is still unknown, the discovery of the effect of ergot has literally been a boon and blessing to thousands of victims of this prostrating affliction. The derivative of ergot used in migraine is

95

ergotamine, and its prime value is in the treatment of acute attacks.

Incidentally it is yet another example of how doctors and patients were using the right form of treatment long before the backroom boys in the research laboratories were able to provide scientific evidence in favour of it. Needless to say, in this interregnum many clever specialists in the Harley Streets of all our medical-school towns were 'pooh-poohing' the poor ignorant general practitioners who knew nothing of what was going on in that rarified atmosphere in which specialists hobnobbed with the scientific elite.

The practice which family doctors and patients had found so useful was to combine ergotamine with caffeine, which, of course, as everyone, or at least nearly everyone, knows, relieves headaches of all sorts. This combination they found more effective than giving ergotamine alone; the caffeine seemed to have an enhancing effect on the ergotamine. So impressed were both doctors and patients with the effectiveness of the combination that the majority of prescriptions in the United Kingdom were for the combined drugs.

Using radioactively labelled compounds, research workers in Basle have now shown that the addition of caffeine to ergotamine leads to a more rapid and effective absorption of ergotamine into the bloodstream, thus enhancing its effect in relieving the headache of migraine. So once again the customer has proved to be right.

A more recent derivative of ergot, known as methysergide, is proving of value in the prevention of migrainous attacks. Unfortunately, it is not without its dangers, and therefore it is only used under strict medical control, and in really severe cases.

'Where ignorance is bliss, 'tis folly to be wise' is an adage that could justifiably be applied to ergot, and borne in mind by the millions of people who have benefited from its use – whether in childbirth or in the throes of migraine. Few, if any, of these beneficiaries are aware that the nucleus of all the alkaloids, or active principles, is a substance known as lysergic acid. That name alone may not ring a bell in every mind, but a derivative of it, lysergic acid diethylamide, or, to be more accurate, its abbreviation, LSD, is now a household word. As Macaulay would have said, every schoolboy knows that this is the most hallucinogenic, or mind-disturbing, drug known to man, but very few probably realized that it is so closely associated with ergot. Indeed, it was only some thirty years ago that, quite accidentally, Swiss research workers stumbled on the fact. This they did because lysergic acid itself proved to be too unstable a substance to be a satisfactory research tool. It was therefore decided to produce what are known as amides of it, as these are much more stable. The story of the discovery of the hallucinogenic action of LSD is one of the most dramatic in the history of therapeutics, and is best told in the words of Dr Albert Hofmann, the Swiss pharmacologist who made the discovery in 1943.

> 'When I was purifying lysergic acid diethylamide I experienced a strange dream-like state which wore off after some hours. The nature and cause of this extraordinary disturbance aroused my suspicions that some exogenic intoxication might be involved and that the substance with which I had been working could be responsible. In order to ascertain whether or not this was so, I decided to test the compound on myself. Being by nature a cautious man, I started my experiment with the lowest dose which presumably could have any effect, taking 0·25 mg. This first planned experiment with LSD took a dramatic turn and led to the discovery of the extraordinarily high psychotomimetic activity of this compound.'

On another occasion he elaborated on this 'dramatic turn':

> 'I was overcome by a fear that I was going out of my mind ... Space and time became more and more disorganized ...

I could do nothing to prevent the breakdown of the world around ... I had a feeling as if I was out of my body. I thought I had died ... I even saw my dead body lying on the sofa.'

In view of the fact that in his ignorance he had taken ten times what is now known to be the usual dose, it is not surprising that Dr Hofmann had such a terrifying experience – an experience that has been repeated all too often in these permissive days when so many members of a civilization in search of God are staging an escape into the unknown by means of LSD.

Not unnaturally, all this aroused the interest of Dr Hofmann and his colleagues in psychotropic drugs, as they are known. This led them to investigate ololiuqui. This is the Aztec name for one of the traditional magic plants of Mexico, *Rivea corymbosa*, which is still used in parts of Mexico for divinatory purposes in medico-mystical practices. They also studied another plant, used by another tribe of Indians for the same purpose, *Ipomoea violacea*, which is none other than the ornamental plant, morning glory, the pride of so many gardens in all parts of the world. In both of these plants they found ergot alkaloids and lysergic acid diethylamide. There are certain structural differences between LSD and the alkaloids of ololiuqui, which result in the latter being much less hallucinogenic than LSD but more narcotic.

When Dr Hofmann's hallucinogenic experience became generally known in Britain after the end of the war, British pharmacologists were naturally interested, though perhaps somewhat sceptical, wondering if perhaps there was, for example, an individual variation in the reaction to LSD. I well recall the late Professor Bain, then Professor of Pharmacology in the University of Leeds, telling me in the late 1940s of his experience with the drug. He had decided to try it out on himself and one or two members of his staff who had been studying it with him. He admitted to me that before his experiment he had wondered whether Dr Hofmann had perhaps exaggerated to a certain extent, and that with a smaller dose the result might not be so cataclysmic. On the other hand, he decided to play for safety and to take it at home. He therefore invited his colleagues to dinner, and after the meal was over the prescribed dose was taken. It was not long before they realized that what Dr Hofmann had described was no exaggeration. Having taken a smaller dose, the hallucinogenic effect was not quite so dramatic, but it was quite dramatic enough to persuade Professor Bain that this was an experiment he was not going to repeat on himself.

In a well-ordered tale this hallucinogenic action of ergot should be the climax of the story, but the logic of time demands a short postscript. As this chapter was being written, an annotation appeared in *The Lancet* about a new derivative of ergot, bromocriptine, which had been introduced into medicine for the suppression of lactation. To stop the maternal breast producing milk is an all too common practice these days, but, apart from doing this simply because the mother does not want to feed her own baby, there are genuine reasons why it must be carried out. As a rule this is achieved by use of one of the sex hormones, often the one known as stilboestrol.

It has been known for some time that ergot derivatives disturbed the hormonal balance in the body necessary for the production of milk from the breast, and this new derivative has been specially synthesized to produce this action. That it is effective is suggested by one trial in sixty patients, in whom it proved as effective for this purpose as stilboestrol. Evidence is also forthcoming that, presumably linked up with its effect on the hormonal balance of the body, it may be of value in the treatment of infertility in women. According to a report from St Bartholomew's Hospital, London, thirteen pregnancies occurred in twelve women treated with bromocriptine for infertility. What is even more intriguing, however, is the suggestion – and at the moment it is no more than a suggestion – that it might prove of value in the treatment of one type of cancer of the breast.

Yet another offshoot of this effect of bromocriptine on the hormonal balance of the body is the possibility of its being of value in the treatment of the enlarged prostate – one of the bugbears of the ageing male, the only known treatment of which at the moment is surgical removal of the enlarged gland. As there is experimental evidence that in animals this enlargement is associated with hormonal disturbances, surgeons have investigated the effect of bromocriptine on enlarged prostates in man, and a preliminary report suggests that this versatile synthetic derivative of ergot may be of value – in some cases at least. As the surgeons concerned cautiously put it: 'A further evaluation of the therapeutic value of this drug on patients with benign prostatic hypertrophy is required.

This, however, is not the end of the story. Evidence is now forthcoming that bromocriptine may have an even wider field of action. The most exciting of these possibilities is that it may be helpful in the treatment of the condition called Parkinsonism or Parkinson's disease after the London general practitioner who first described it, but still popularly known as paralysis agitans. This is a disease characterized by tremulousness of the hands, stiffness of the legs leading to difficulty in walking, difficulty in talking and eating, and a pathetic expressionless face. It is mainly an affliction of the elderly, in whom it can cause untold misery. Fortunately, in recent years several new drugs have been discovered which help in controlling the condition and thus make life more bearable for these unfortunate senior citizens.

A report from University College Hospital, London, based on the results with bromocriptine in twelve patients with Parkinsonism, refers to 'striking improvement' in the majority, with complete failure in only one. Not the least important aspect of this report is that bromocriptine proved of value in patients who had not responded to other drugs used for the condition or could not tolerate them. Granted that this is only a preliminary report on a small number of patients but, coming from one of our leading teaching hospitals, it holds out high hopes of ergot extending even farther afield its service to mankind.

Such then is the treasure box provided for us by Nature in the form, not of a herb, but of a much more lowly form of growth – a fungus, which lives on a herb. It is not only an example of a 'herb' that heals; it is also an example of how the research laboratory can contribute to the benefit of suffering humanity by an intensive study of the products of Nature. In making such a study, however, the research worker must never ignore tradition. If he does, then there occurs such disgraceful stories as the use of ergot in midwifery. On the other hand, always bearing tradition in mind – whether that of 'old wives' tales' or that of the practising doctor – the research worker can often, as in the case of ergot, discover drugs and remedies which would otherwise never have seen the light of day.

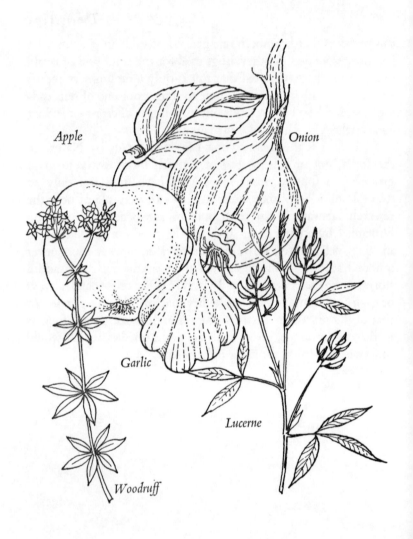

Apple

Onion

Garlic

Lucerne

Woodruff

7

To clot or not to clot

In 1921, cattle in the cattle-rearing state of North Dakota and the neighbouring province of Ontario started bleeding to death. In some cases the bleeding was spontaneous, leading to death in a matter of a few hours. In others it followed some form of trauma – often quite minor. Thus, in one herd of eighty calves, sixty-five died of haemorrhage following dehorning, while in another incident twelve out of twenty-five young bulls bled to death following castration. Typical of what tended to happen is the episode described by one veterinary pathologist of the farmer who, 'following the traditions of his elders, cut a slice of skin and cartilage from the ears of all his yearling cattle and then retired for the night. This was to have had the mysterious effect of a blood tonic.' It was a much more 'mysterious' effect when he came down the next morning and found his yearlings bleeding profusely. The application of ligatures saved them from immediate death, but they all succumbed to haemorrhage within a few weeks. Even more sinister was the heavy death roll among calving cows, both cow and calf often dying of haemorrhage.

Because of the economic importance of the disease it was

quickly referred for investigation to the experts at the Ontario Veterinary College and the Agricultural Experimental Station of North Dakota. They soon established that this was a hitherto unknown disease, no record of which could be found in veterinary archives. The first reaction of both farmers and vets was to blame it on sweet clover which had recently been introduced as a new fodder crop. For a conservative section of the community such as farmers who – often rightly – tend to be suspicious of innovations, this was an entirely natural reaction. On the other hand, being so dependent on the vagaries of Nature, they are an observant breed, the most successful of whom acquire what can best be described as an affinity with Nature that often seems – at least to the town-lubber – to verge on second sight. Whether this is true of the mechanized farmer of today is another matter.

Be that as it may, the farmers of North Dakota proved to be right, and the investigators tracked the cause of this new disease – henceforth to be known as sweet clover disease, or toxic sweet clover disease – to the eating of spoiled sweet clover resulting from faulty curing. A simple experiment, as detailed in the extensive summary of the investigators' findings, is typical of the overwhelming evidence produced in favour of this conclusion.

'Good clover stalks and damaged clover stalks were picked from the same hay mow. The good were fed to one rabbit and the damaged to another. The rabbit which ate the good remained well, while the rabbit which ate the bad died, showing typical haemorrhagic lesions. This experiment was duplicated, using a different sample of clover hay. The results were the same.'

Thus was the first hurdle – and from the farmers' point of view the most important – cleared. The bleeding was due to spoiled sweet clover and could therefore be prevented by not allowing cattle to eat such diseased hay. This still left, however, the problem of how the bleeding was brought about. The first reaction was that it was due to the moulds that spoiled the sweet clover – again a perfectly natural reaction. But this proved to be a false clue, and it was not until 1941, after a period of twenty years' intensive research, that the toxic factor was finally tracked down, synthesized, and given the name of dicoumarol.

This name it owes to the fact that it is a derivative of coumarin, which gives the characteristic odour to new-mown hay. It is present in around 150 species of plants, including woodruff and tonco beans. The latter, which are the dried seeds of a large tree growing in Brazil, Venezuela and Guyana, are the main commercial source of coumarin, which is used in perfumery and in tobacco manufacture though, today, synthetic coumarin is tending to replace the natural substance. It is its coumarin content that has given woodruff its popularity from pre-Christian days. One of its most widespread uses was for flavouring wine, it being the basis, for instance, of the well-known hock-cup, maibowle or maitrank. Its characteristic smell also made it one of the so-called strewing herbs scattered on the floors of mansions, baronial and otherwise, as an antidote to the stench of unwashed humanity in the old days. It was also used in linen chests on account of its coumarin odour, while in the Netherlands it was used for stuffing beds – a pleasing idea that some enterprising modern rural hotelier might profitably revive. Medicinally, it acquired a wide reputation in the Middle Ages as a blood purifier.

The clotting of blood is one of the most complicated processes in the body. Indeed, it is only now that we are beginning to appreciate its complexity. It is, of course, one of the essential functions of the body for the simple reason that, if our blood did not clot then, like the bovine victims of sweet clover disease, we would bleed to death. Dicoumarol interferes with this process by depressing the production in the liver of several of the factors responsible for clotting, including prothrombin. This it does by a clever piece of subterfuge, the elucidation of which requires a switch from North America to Denmark.

While the Americans were investigating sweet clover disease, two Danish research workers described in 1934 a nutritional disease in chickens characterized by bleeding. The first thought was that this was a form of scurvy due to lack of vitamin C, but this was soon disproved. On the other hand, it could be prevented by giving the chickens a variety of foodstuffs, particularly lucerne or decayed fish meal. Lucerne, or alfalfa, of course, is one of the major forage crops of the world, with a reputation for increasing the quality and yield of milk, and also one of the oldest, having been used by the Medes and Persians. It contains a range of vitamins, but not vitamin C, and is one of the commercia sources of chlorophyll. Human nature being what it is, with a reputation and constitution such as this, it was inevitable that it should be tried out on man, and for a time an infusion of alfalfa, to be taken before meals, enjoyed a reputation for increasing vitality, appetite and weight.

The Danish workers finally isolated the active principle in alfalfa and other foodstuffs which prevented bleeding, and, in 1935, named it vitamin K (Koagulations-vitamin). Four years later it was synthesized, and is now the possessor, in the *Pharmacopoieas* of the world of the complicated name of phytomenadione. It is fairly widespread in Nature: in dark-green vegetables such as kale and spinach, and nettles, as well as alfalfa. Cauliflower is also a good source, as are pine needles.

The precise *modus operandi* of vitamin K in preventing bleeding is still not quite clear, but it is known that it is an essential ingredient of the enzyme in the liver which is responsible for producing prothrombin and the other clotting factors, whose production is prevented or depressed by dicoumarol. If this enzyme is not present and functioning properly, then clotting is prevented and bleeding occurs on the slightest provocation (or trauma, in technical terms). And here comes the subterfuge referred to. The chemical structure of dicoumarol is similar to that of vitamin K. This means that, if the body is flooded with dicoumarol the enzyme in the liver responsible for the production of the clotting factors mistakes it for vitamin K and absorbs it into its structure. By so doing it loses the ability to sponsor the production of the clotting factors, and just to make sure that this fell purpose is properly achieved, it is unable to incorporate vitamin K when it comes along. Thus, rather like the cuckoo in the nest, if you like, dicoumarol plays a deceitful role and prevents the essential enzyme performing its function.

Dicoumarol is by no means the only example of this form of subterfuge. It is also the technique followed by the sulphonamides. They are structurally similar to a substance known as PABA (para-amino-benzoic acid, to give it its full title) which is essential for the survival of certain bacteria. This means that the enzyme in the bacteria responsible for coping with PABA and converting it into the substances, or metabolites, essential to their metabolism, is deceived by the sulphonamides, lap them up and then find they are unable to cope with PABA – with the resultant death of the bacteria from inanition. It is a technique that was in due course developed by investigators of new drugs and is now used in designing and synthesizing drugs.

The happy sequel of the sweet clover disease story is that dicoumarol, along with other coumarin derivatives, soon came to play a valuable part in controlling the clotting of blood that can prove so dangerous a complication in various diseases such as, for example, thrombophlebitis, and the killing form of clotting known as pulmonary embolism. These anticoagulants, as they are known, are among the most important drugs in our therapeutic armamentarium today; they also occur, incidentally, in the form of Warfarin, a most efficient rat poison – or rodenticide to use modern jargon.

It is an eminently satisfying conclusion to the investigation of what at the time threatened to be a most serious interference with a major 'industry', one of the major sources of meat for human consumption. Like ergot, the beneficial factor may not have been a herb, but it was so closely linked with one that it is fully entitled to inclusion in this survey of herbs that heal.

From blood clotting to heart disease and high blood pressure may seem a long jump, and when it is suggested that the gap may be bridged by means of onions and garlic, the eyebrows of even the most accommodating of readers have some excuse for being raised. The association, however, is not merely one of ideas, and is not in reality as far fetched as it seems. The technical background to all this is just about as complicated as it could be, but can be briefly summarized without the sacrifice of too much accuracy.

It is not only necessary to prevent clotting of blood in the body. It is also necessary for the body to remove clots when they do develop. This means not only the larger clots which occasionally occur and cause so much trouble. It also involves the minute clots which form quite often, but of which we are entirely unaware. As these 'mini' episodes involve fibrin, the essential constituent of a clot, the process of disposing of them is known as fibrino-lysis – or the lysis (or breaking down) of fibrin – and the drugs that are used to facilitate this process are known as fibrinolytic drugs. This is all fairly straightforward in theory – if highly complicated in practice – but there is evidence that fibrinolytic agents have also an effect on the lipid, or fatty, contents of the blood and even on some of the proteins in the blood. The significance of this in the present context is that there is some correlation between the concentration of certain blood lipids, including cholesterol, and the incidence of disease of the walls of the arteries: it is this disease, or arteriosclerosis as it is technically known, that is associated with coronary heart disease, which is such a common cause of death today, and also of strokes and high blood pressure. And now to our onions and garlic.

The modern version of the story begins in 1968 when an article by a team of Indian doctors, entitled 'Effect of Onions on Blood Fibrinolytic Activity', appeared in the *British Medical Journal*, with the following introductory paragraph: 'A casual remark by a patient that in France, when a horse develops clots in the legs, it is treated by a diet of garlic and onions led one of us to investigate onions as a possible source of a fibrinolytic agent.' They went on to report that the addition of onions, either fried or boiled, to what is described as the fat-enriched breakfast of patients, not only prevented the decrease in fibrinolytic activity of the blood that normally follows such a high-fat diet, but actually increased fibrinolysis.

The interest of this observation lay in the fact that it was known that in certain parts of India, such as Rajasthan, where most of the population take onions as a major part of their diet, the incidence of coronary heart disease is lower than among those who do not eat onions for some religious reason. The question therefore arose whether this was sheer coincidence or whether the addition of onions to the diet might have some protective value against the development of that form of arterial disease that leads to coronary heart disease, by virtue of this increase in the fibrinolytic activity of the blood. Subsequent work, all carried out on patients or volunteers, indicated that the addition of onions to the high-fat type of diet which normally results in an increase in the amount of lipids in the blood, prevented this rise in blood lipids as well as preventing the decrease in fibrinolytic activity induced by a high-fat diet. There was also some evidence that this effect of onions was more marked in older, than younger, patients.

An experiment has also been reported in rabbits, in which arteriosclerosis can be induced fairly easily by giving them cholesterol. In this experiment, involving forty rabbits, the addition of onions to their diet did not lower the level of cholesterol in the blood when extra cholesterol was given, or prevent the development of arteriosclerosis, whereas garlic achieved both these aims. Granted that it is notoriously dangerous to attempt to translate the effects on cholesterol metabolism in rabbits into what happens in human beings but, taken in conjunction with experiments carried out in patients and volunteers, and the apparent correlation between the taking of onions and the incidence of coronary heart disease, these findings are certainly worthy of further consideration.

Before reviewing the historical background, against which these current observations must be viewed in order to maintain a correct sense of perspective, two further developments in our knowledge of the effects of onions and garlic must be mentioned. Some twenty years ago reports began appearing in the Indian medical journals of both onions and garlic lowering the concentration of sugar in the blood of both normal people and those with diabetes. Within the last couple of years a further series of reports to the same effect have appeared; this time attempting to track down and isolate the factor, or principle, responsible for this action which might well be of value in the treatment of diabetes. Typical of these is one in which the action of onion juice and of garlic on the blood-sugar level in rabbits after they had been given a large amount of glucose was compared with that of tolbutamide, a drug used in the treatment of diabetes, and water. The results showed that the maximal percentage fall in the blood sugar was 1·8 with water, 7.1 with onion juice, 12·4 with garlic and 19·6 with tolbutamide.

The significance of these observations is that there is a close correlation between diabetes and arterial disease, just as there is a considerable amount of evidence linking coronary disease with a high consumption of sugar. Is there a possibility that, by virtue of their combined action on blood lipids, blood sugar and fibrinolytic activity of the blood, onions and garlic may prove of value in the treatment or prevention of coronary heart disease – the major killing disease of Western civilization in the current era?

Closely associated with that form of arterial disease known as arteriosclerosis, though not synonymous with it, is high blood pressure (or hypertension as it is known), another affliction of modern life. Whether it is a new phenomenon is debatable as it is only within the last hundred years that we have been able to measure the blood pressure in patients, and in any case far more people are surviving to the age when the blood pressure naturally tends to rise in some people. Be all that as it may, it is such a common condition today that any safe and effective way of keeping it under control cannot be ignored. Hence the more than passing interest of an Indian doctor's letter in *The Lancet* in 1969, in which he reported that he had obtained promising results from the use of garlic in five consecutive patients with high blood pressure, and that he was planning a controlled trial of it in a further series of cases. As no further report had been published by the summer of 1975, I wrote to him and asked him whether he had ever been able to undertake such a trial. To this letter he replied:

'The trial had to be dropped since I could not get extracts of garlic for further trials. First I gave crude powdered extract of garlic to patients with hypertension which gave me very encouraging results. I tried this remedy for hypertension because in this part of the country, Southern Madras, they give garlic to pregnant women from the second trimester of pregnancy and these women do not suffer from tox-aemia of pregnancy. [This is a complication of pregnancy accompanied by high blood pressure.]

Because of these observations I wanted to do a scientific study, and did a provisional trial with the crude substance, but I could not proceed further with a controlled trial because of lack of facilities in Madras in isolating the active principle from garlic.'

Such then is the modern history of onions and garlic. What about their past? This dates right back into the earliest days. The onion, indigenous to Asia, is said to be one of the oldest cultivated vegetables. Certainly it was held in high esteem in ancient Egypt, and references are found to it in the records of all the ancient civilizations. One of the many claims made for it in the Middle Ages was that it was good for the growth of hair. Perhaps its major reputation, however, was as an antiseptic, and well into this century in certain parts of the country an esteemed method of bringing boils and carbuncles to a head was a poultice made of onions and black treacle. It also had a reputation as an expectorant, and as a diuretic to increase the flow of urine, but for this latter purpose it was often given along with gin, to which the diuretic action must be attributed. Applied externally it was a popular remedy for unbroken chilblains and wasp and bee stings. Recurrently it surfaces as a remedy for insomnia, taken either boiled or baked. I well recall two delightful maiden aunts of mine, who were anything but hypochondriacs or food faddists, having a passing craze for onions for the good of their health – more or less on the principle that an onion a day kept the doctor away.

Garlic, however, has always been higher up in the medical hierarchy, only being finally removed from the *British Pharmaceutical Codex* as recently as 1954, and it still features in the French and Spanish *Pharmacopoieias*. According to *Martindale*, the wise doctor's *vade-mecum* in such matters, it has 'expectorant, diaphoretic, disinfectant and diuretic properties' and has 'been used as a syrup in chronic bronchitis'. In ancient days it had much more glowing testimonials, though Horace deplored its use, as did Maimonides, the famous Jewish physician of the twelfth century.

The Romans had such a high opinion of it that they dedicated it to Mars and to encourage their legionaries to eat it and so enhance their courage, they propagated it wherever they went – thus introducing it, incidentally, to Britain. Dioscorides, Nero's physician, recommended it for a more peaceful purpose: mixed with sugar to clear the voice, a practice still followed by operatic tenors in France and Italy, to the discomfiture, as often as not, of their singing opposite numbers.

Like onions, it has an age-old reputation as an antiseptic and cleanser of the body. It was used both internally and externally in the treatment of rheumatism, and not uncommonly the bruised bulbs mixed with lard were rubbed on the chest of the unfortunate child with whooping-cough. Syrupus Allii, a mixture of garlic and sugar, was at one time a popular remedy for chronic bronchitis, and for many a long year country folk in England swore that tuberculosis could be cured by eating raw garlic every day. Interestingly enough, towards the end of the last war, that is, just before the introduction of PAS and streptomycin, reports emanated from Russia that promising results were being obtained in the later stages of tuberculosis from the use of an extract of garlic.

In none of this is there any suggestion that either onions or garlic might prove of value in controlling the state of health of our arteries, unless its reputation among the Roman legionaries could be linked up in this way. On the other hand, there is the Indian reputation of garlic preventing the onset of high blood pressure in pregnant women, and the veterinary story of its use in the treatment of clots in horses.

Just to round off the story of the possible value of herbs in helping to control arteriosclerosis, with all its dire consequences, and also to show that it is not only in the East that this problem is being tackled, comes a report that appeared in *The Lancet* as this chapter was being planned. It came from the Gastroenterology

Unit of the Medical Research Council, and showed that two products of the plant world cause significant falls in the level of cholesterol in the blood. One of these is guar gum, or guar flour, which comes from the seeds of the cluster bean (*Cyamopsis tetragonolobus*), the main use of which in the West is as a thickening agent in sauces and an emulsion stabilizer, though it is also sold as an appetite suppressant. The other is pectin, which comes from apples and for centuries has been used as a gelling agent in making jam. While both guar gum and pectin were found to lower the blood cholesterol levels, wheat fibre, or bran, tended to raise them.

The conclusion of this report admirably epitomizes the scope of the problem facing us in this field and stresses the necessity for a new, non-drug approach, an approach in which healing herbs have obviously an important part to play.

This conclusion is that 'this work emphasizes the importance of "natural" substances in lowering the serum cholesterol at a time when dietary fibre – which has become synonymous with wheat bran – has been shown to have no effect in the short term. Perhaps we should look at the diets eaten in those parts of the world from which many of our epidemiological clues have come. Wheat fibre is of little nutritional relevance in many parts of Asia and Africa where rice, vegetables and fruit are staple foods. Low-fat intake is recognized as an important factor in maintaining low cholesterol levels. Increased consumption of gel-containing vegetables and fruits may be yet another.' As a postscript they note that patents have been taken out on a wide range of natural gels and mucilages, all of which have been shown to have a cholesterol-lowering effect.

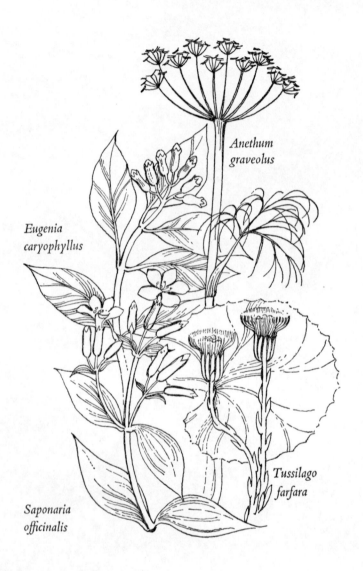

Anethum
graveolus

Eugenia
caryophyllus

Saponaria
officinalis

Tussilago
farfara

8
Spices, coughs and colds

Without spices the culinary art could not exist. They have been an integral part of the dietetic habits of mankind since time immemorial. Originally used to disguise the taste and smell of malodorous rotting flesh, they gradually assumed the more sophisticated role of stimulating the flagging appetites of those members of society who, with more money than sense, overgorged themselves, and had to have their appetites artificially stimulated in order to sit down and enjoy the next meal. By a relatively early stage in the so-called civilizing process therefore spices had become definitely 'U', in the Mitfordian terminology of the 1950s, a snob value actively encouraged by the spicers of those and subsequent days, with the result that their price soared to relatively astronomical heights.

In due course therefore they became a stimulant to empire building, as well as to appetite building, and 'India's spicy shores' and 'the spicy shore of Araby the blest' from the days of the Arab ascendancy onwards became the naval battlegrounds of the world. Later, from the fifteenth century onwards, European predators stepped in: first the Portuguese, then the Dutch and finally the

British. Each in turn tried to create a monopoly for each spice, whether in India, Ceylon, or the islands of the East Indies or the Indian Ocean, not hesitating to destroy all the spice plants in other islands to ensure that the monopoly should be retained intact. How much of the wealth of the East India Company, for instance, came from these shiploads of spices which they brought to England?

Alcoholic liquors, too, were laced with spice, both wine and beer. Milton's 'spicy nut-brown ale' was the popular drink of his day and for many a long year afterwards. Gradually, as the standards of brewing improved, particularly after the introduction of hops into the process, the spices became 'non-U', just as they did in wines, so that today it is only in liqueurs and aperitifs that they figure to any extent. In them, of course, they are the essential ingredients apart from the alcohol, and the spices give them their distinctive flavour as, for instance, caraway in kümmel and cloves in plum and cherry brandy.

Medicinally they have almost as old a record, naturally starting with the ancient Chinese and Hindu civilizations, and then gradually coming westwards during the great imperial days of Persia, Egypt, Greece and Rome. The claims made for them were often reminiscent of the quack herbalists of yesteryear, but on analysis they boil down to the one dominating claim that they soothed the gut. This was followed by a host of secondary claims, the most important of which were for coughs and colds, and as the basis for soothing, sedative hot drinks, interestingly enough, often for mother and child.

This is of more than passing interest when one comes to compare this list with what the current edition of *Martindale*, published by direction of the Council of the Pharmaceutical Society of Great Britain, and justifiably described on the dust-cover as 'the authoritative reference work on drugs and medicines in current use', has to say about them. The active ingredients of spices are the so-called essential oils, and no better brief account of their medicinal attributes could be found than that provided by *Martindale*. Taken internally, they act as restoratives in the case of syncope, as mild expectorants (or easers of the coughing up of sputum) and as carminatives, being 'employed for the relief of gastric discomfort and of flatulent colic'. Applied externally to the unbroken skin they act as counter-irritants 'in the treatment of chronic inflammatory conditions, and to relieve neuralgia and rheumatic pains'. Finally, 'when inhaled they render secretions more fluid and relieve congestion of the bronchioles and they may be employed for this purpose in conditions such as chronic bronchitis'.

It is not proposed to elaborate to any extent on this sober summing up of the current medicinal attributes of these spices of old. It may sound plebeian when matched against memories of the clove-drenched atmosphere of Zanzibar, or even one's childhood memories of the old-fashioned chemist's shop, or – a joy in store for those who have not yet experienced it – the pleasingly aromatic atmosphere of the reconstructed seventeenth century pharmacy in the Shambles in York. On the other hand it presents the case for preserving these herbs that heal in this modern age. It is a case that is often criticized by the advocates of today's synthetic drugs; this is particularly so in the case of their use as carminatives and bitters – two terms, incidentally, that the scientific doctors of today would like to see abolished simply, it would appear, because they do not fit nicely into the 'new look' of scientific medicine. Medicine, however, is an art as well as a science, and even the most cursory glance at the functions of carminatives and bitters will show that they still have a useful function to subserve in the practice of medicine.

Carminatives are preparations to relieve flatulence and any resulting griping by the bringing up of wind. Their precise mode of action is still rather obscure but in practice, when swallowed, they induce a pleasant taste in the mouth which may be accompanied by an increased flow of saliva. This is followed by a sensation of warmth as they are swallowed, and sooner or later there follows the bringing up of wind. Practically any spices will achieve this, the most commonly used being caraway, cardamom, cinnamon, cloves, dill, ginger, nutmeg and peppermint. In this way they can undoubtedly help people to renew their interest in food and thereby increase, or at least restore, their interest in life. Whether or not this is accompanied by the bringing up of wind is actually incidental, though there are few males of the species who do not derive a considerable degree of satisfaction from a good old-fashioned belch.

Bitters are among the oldest of drugs still prescribed, and include a wide range extending beyond that of spices. Wormwood, probably the oldest of them all, is mentioned in the Ebers papyrus (1500 BC), but is never prescribed today. It is, of course, with aniseed, one of the constituents of absinthe, a form of alcoholic liquor that had to be banned by the French during the 1914–18 War because of the devastatingly demoralizing effect it was having on the soldiery. Bitters are referred to in the Hippocratic writings of around 400 BC and have been defined as 'alcoholic extracts of herbs used to stimulate the diet and to a lesser extent a flavouring for tonics and other remedies'. They have been subdivided into three categories – *simple bitters*, used to stimulate appetite and the action of the stomach, and including calumba and gentian; *aromatic bitters*, which combine the property of bitterness with that of aromatic volatile oils, and are used as carminatives; and *incidental bitters*, in which the bitter function is incidental to more important therapeutic effects. Among the herbal members of this group are quinine and strychnine.

As in the case of carminatives, the precise mode of action of bitters is not clear, but they are known to increase gastric secretion and thereby often have a beneficial effect by improving the individual's interest in food. Granted that the wise thing is to try and find out the cause of the loss of appetite and remove this. Often, however, this is not possible and even when it is, removal of the cause may not restore the appetite. It is in these circumstances that the wise family doctor prescribes bitters, fully appreciating that in some cases the beneficial effect may be psychological; but what does that matter so long as appetite is restored?

Of all the carminative spices perhaps the best known today is dill, the dried ripe fruit of *Anethum graveolens*, which is indigenous to southern Europe. Its name is derived from the Norse *dilla*, to soothe, on account of its reputation as a soothing herb. It is one of the many herbs mentioned in Egyptian papyri, and there are records of its use in England since Anglo-Saxon days. It was at one time a popular remedy for hiccups, and recipes for dill tea are still to be found with earnest commendations in popular herbal treatises. Its main claim to medicinal fame today, however, is in the form of dill water, a prescription for which is still provided in the *British Pharmaceutical Codex*, with a note that 'Dill Water is a carminative used in the treatment of flatulence in infants.' Indeed, there must be relatively few 'windy infants' who have not at some time or other had their 'burbulence' relieved by this traditional remedy.

Of those spices which relieve and ease congested air passages when inhaled, probably the best known is eucalyptus, or eucalyptus oil to give it its full title. One of its constituents, eucalyptol, has antimicrobial properties, on the basis of which it is included in some dentifrices, and along with zinc oxide it is used as a temporary dental filling. It is the oil which over the years has been widely used for the relief of aching throats, stuffy noses and blocked bronchial tubes. For this reason it still retains its place in the *British Pharmacopoeia*. Its attributes in this sphere are concisely but aptly summarized by the *British Pharmaceutical Codex*, according to which:

'To relieve cough in chronic bronchitis and asthma it is inhaled from steam, sometimes with the addition of menthol, pine oil, and compound benzoin tincture. It is an ingredient of pastilles, often with menthol, for the symptomatic relief of the common cold.'

These self-same pastilles, or lozenges, are also often sucked as a protection against infection. To some this may appear somewhat anti-social in public places, as it is not everyone who appreciates the smell of this particular spice. On the other hand, even though the antimicrobial activity of the contained eucalyptus may not be sufficient to suggest that this gives any real protection against infection, it is a fairly harmless (and cheap) custom, which may give some psychological protection to the nervous citizen travelling in crowded buses or underground trains at the height of the 'common cold' season, and the psychological factor in infection is not to be ignored. In addition, the odour is no more anti-social than many of the other odours humanity carries about with it, such as garlic. Yet another popular use of eucalyptus at one time was to sprinkle it on one's handkerchief or pillow. For the solitary sleeper the latter is certainly a useful method of clearing the stuffy nose on going to bed and so encouraging more rapid sleep.

Eucalyptus also illustrates one of the other therapeutic activities of the essential oils: namely, that of relieving neuralgic or rheumatic pains. For this purpose it is applied in the form of an ointment, liniment or embrocation. One domestic remedy of this type used to be an embrocation of equal parts of eucalyptus oil and olive oil. For some skins this might be rather too potent, and the medical prescription used to be a liniment containing 25% of the eucalyptus oil.

One could go on almost indefinitely in this fascinating world of the spices, but one more must be mentioned before the subject is changed, because of the increasing attention it is receiving as a manipulator of the mind.

Nutmeg comes from the dried seeds of *Myristica fragrans*, an evergreen aromatic tree indigenous to the Molucca Islands, but now widely cultivated in Indonesia, Malaysia, Sri Lanka and Grenada. So potent at times is its characteristic aromatic odour that it is said that in the 'Spice Isles' of the East Indies, as they are known, the birds of paradise fall to the ground overcome by the aroma. Originally introduced into the Levant by the Arabs in the twelfth century, it soon found its way into Europe where it proved so popular that, when the Portuguese in the fifteenth century discovered the Banda Islands in the East Indies, where the tree grew profusely, they immediately established a monopoly, to be ousted in due course by the Dutch. This monopoly was not broken until the end of the eighteenth century when for a short time the British occupied the Spice Isles, and immediately trans- planted some of the trees to Penang and elsewhere in Malaya, so breaking the Dutch monopoly once and for all.

Today the main interest lies in the psychotropic or mental action of several of its constituents, including myristicin. Although one sixteenth century herbal did refer to its 'cleansing the brain of superfluous humours', this claim was so mixed up with the other stock ones made for spices, such as clearing the wind, and 'taking away the offensive fumes of a strong breath', that little attention was paid to it. It was not until the earlier stages of the current craze for probing into the mind-stimulating activities of every drug, new and old alike, that it began to be realized that nutmeg was a 'winner' in this respect.

Needless to say, the inmates of USA prisons were early on to its possibilities, and their eggnogs well besprinkled with grated nutmeg soon became a popular 'kick'. Quite independently, one or two harassed housewives in the USA discovered that the regular consumption of grated nutmeg from the larder took the edge off life, and in due course this percolated through to the medical profession. After inevitable initial disbelief on the part of the 'pukka' members of the profession, the light dawned: the outcome of the subsequent investigation was that, by virtue predominantly of the myristicin they contained, nutmegs produced a psychedelic state characterized by visual illusions, feelings of unreality, levitation and isolation. This was not surprising when it was noted that the chemical structure of myristicin was similar to that of mescaline and amphetamine.

More recent work has indicated that myristicin may not be the only factor in nutmegs responsible for these psychotic or hallucinogenic activities. That, however, is a technical point, and what continuing research is bringing forth is evidence that factors in nutmegs have a widespread effect on what is known as the sympathetic nervous system of the body, and that they may also antagonize the action of prostaglandins which are proving to be among the most important constituents of the body. Knowledge of the prostaglandins has accumulated so rapidly, and their activity is proving so versatile, playing a part, for instance, in such variegated actions as childbirth, the evocation of pain, the constriction of the bronchi in asthma, and the disturbance of the bowels responsible for diarrhoea, that no concise summary of their precise role can yet be given. What is proven, however, and what is relevant if nutmeg can affect the activity of at least some of them, is that a vast new field is opening up for the possible role of this age-old plant that heals.

An interesting example of the new role of nutmeg as an antagonist to prostaglandins comes from California. A seventy-one-year-old man developed diarrhoea. Recalling that powdered nutmeg was sometimes given to cattle to control diarrhoea, he started to take a teaspoonful of it four times a day and found that this promptly relieved the diarrhoea. In due course he was treated by the medical profession who investigated the cause of the diarrhoea, and one of the first things the doctors did was to 'try more traditional approaches to therapy', but 'with incomplete relief'. The patient was therefore allowed to go back to his nutmeg which once again did the trick and continued to do so until he died some three years later. The point of this case history is that the final conclusion was that the diarrhoea in this man was due to an abnormal overproduction of a certain prostaglandin, and that the powdered nutmeg worked by antagonizing this excess.

A close and traditional competitor of the essential oils of spices as alleviators of the discomforts of coughs and colds is the group of plant derivatives known as balsams, which contain various resins. The most widely used of these is benzoin, a balsamic resin derived from the incised stem of *Styrax benzoin*, a tree cultivated in Sumatra. It is best known as one of the constituents of friars' balsam, or compound benzoin tincture to give it its official title in the *British Pharmaceutical Codex*. While it is occasionally taken internally as an expectorant to loosen the cough in chronic bronchitis, its main use, as every experienced housewife knows, is as an inhalation to clear the air passages and make breathing easier for sufferers with bronchitis, sore throats, laryngitis, and the common cold. It is also applied undiluted, as an antiseptic and to arrest bleeding, to small cuts; yet another use is to apply it to intact skin as a protective dressing under occlusive plasters and bandages. In all of these functions it provides a most useful remedial agent and one which we could ill afford to lose.

Its origin and its name are wrapped in mystery. The earliest reference to a formula resembling the modern one (benzoin, aloes, Tolu balsam and storax) dates back to that of Pomet in the seventeenth century. His formula included benzoin, aloes, Peru balsam, storax, frankincense, myrrh, angelica root and St John's wort flowers. With the exception of aloes, these are all herbs as widely encountered in incense as in medicine, which strongly suggests that balsam is of ecclesiastical origin. Storax, for instance, was commended by the Emperor Constantine to the Church of Rome, and was being used in the churches and mosques of Asia Minor in the latter part of the last century. Further evidence in support of the ecclesiastical origin of the name is that at one time alternative names were Catholic balsam and Jesuits' drops.

Of the other three balsams still in use, two, Peru balsam and Tolu balsam, come from trees indigenous to South America. They owe their names to the fact that the former was originally exported to Spain through Peru, while the latter originally came from around Tolu in Colombia. The third, storax, is from a tree indigenous to Turkey. As already noted, both Tolu balsam and storax are included in friars' balsam, having a comparable action to that of benzoin. Tolu balsam is also widely used in the form of Tolu syrup to flavour cough mixtures. Peru balsam, with equal parts of castor oil, is used for bed-sores and chronic ulcers, and is also incorporated in some suppositories for haemorrhoids.

There is yet another large group of herbs traditionally used for the relief of coughs and bronchial congestion: these are now known to act by virtue of the fact that they have a demulcent or soothing action, often combined with a detergent action. They have this last effect due to the fact that they contain what are known as saponins. These are substances characterized by the property of imparting to water the faculty of frothing: hence their name from the Latin *sapo* (soap). This detergent, or soap-like, property is obviously of great value in loosening the excess secretions which collect in the throat and bronchial passages of the lungs, often in a very tenacious state, and render breathing difficult since they block the entry of air into the lungs. They can also act as an irritant, thereby producing that unproductive, irritating, hacking cough that can prove so exhausting to the ill patient. Saponins also act reflexly by stimulating the lining membrane of the stomach and thereby evoking a reflex of increased production of mucus in the bronchial tubes. This automatically loosens the mucus secretion and allows it to be coughed up more effectively and easily.

With our antibiotics and sulphonamides we can now often get to the root of the problem and eliminate the infection that is responsible for all this, but this is not always possible, as in the case of so many of these virus infections, such as influenza, against which no known drug is yet effective. In such cases therefore the relief of the patient's discomfort, and the lessening of unnecessary strain by easing the cough is fundamentally sound treatment, just as it is in a more secondary way by tiding over the patient receiving antibiotics until these have knocked out the causative micro-organisms.

A comparable soothing or demulcent effect, though produced in a different way, is obtained from the use of herbs containing mucilage; while others prove useful in congested states of the throat and larynx by virtue of the tannin which they contain. By these three different methods, two or more of which may be combined, a large number of traditional herbal remedies for coughs and the like have now been shown to justify their age-old reputation. To list them would be tiresome, but one or two may be picked out as samples of some of the better known herbs that heal in this category.

Perhaps pride of place should be given to soapwort (*Saponaria officinalis*), whose very name, and range of names, such as soap-root, latherwort, and craw soap, indicate its soap-like propensities. In the days when children were satisfied with the simple things of life, and could derive more enjoyment from such simple things than their modern counterparts do from the most sophisticated and expensive toys, a favourite game was to see how much foam one could produce by shaking the leaves of soapwort in water. Soapwort is said to have been introduced to Britain by the Romans, and there is evidence that they utilized its water-softening properties. Medicinally it has had a variegated claim to fame as a remedy for many of the ills of life, including venereal disease – a claim that was probably based on the fact that it has a diuretic effect. In more recent times, its main claim to recognition is as an expectorant and loosener of coughs.

Another saponin-containing herb which has had a long reputation as an expectorant is senega (*Polygala senega*), also known as snakeroot and milkwort. The former name it owes to the fact that among the Indians of North America, where it is indigenous, it had a reputation as a cure for snake bites. In the eighteenth century it attracted the attention of Dr Tennent, an immigrant Scottish doctor. He found it of value in the treatment of pleurisy and pneumonia, and in due course introduced it to the United Kingdom, where it still finds a place in the *British Pharmaceutical Codex* as an expectorant. It owes this reputation to the saponins it contains, which act by stimulating the stomach and thereby inducing an increased secretion of mucus in the bronchial tubes.

Coltsfoot, whose official name, *Tussilago farfara*, indicates its cough-easing properties, and which is also known as coughwort, finally disappeared from the *British Pharmaceutical Codex* in 1949. It still retains, however, its popularity as a domestic cough remedy or, in more technical language, as a 'demulcent to relieve irritating cough', not only in Britain but also in China. The demulcent, or soothing, action is due to the mucilage it contains. It can claim a history going back to the days of Dioscorides in the first century AD. Coltsfoot tea sweetened with honey, taken hot first thing in the morning, is a homely, comforting start to the day for the individual with a troublesome irritating cough. It also has a traditional reputation as a constituent of herbal tobacco for the relief of asthma. This reputation was presumably responsible for the crews of isolated anti-aircraft batteries during the 1939–45 War cultivating it on the site and smoking it instead of more conventional tobacco.

Another herb with a high content of mucilage (up to 30%), and a correspondingly high reputation as a cough soother, is the marshmallow (*Althaea officinalis*). Ever since the days of Theophrastus (380–286 BC), who prescribed grated root of marshmallow for the alleviation of a cough, it has retained its reputation in this respect, only finally disappearing from the *British Pharmaceutical Codex* some twenty years ago. It is still retained in some eighteen *Pharmacopoeias*, many of them including a syrup of marshmallow for sore throats and bronchitis.

Yet another group of herbs useful in the treatment of troublesome throats and larynxes is that containing herbs possessing tannin, which therefore have an astringent action on what are commonly known as relaxed throats. This is a condition liable to afflict those who make their living with their voice such as clergymen, actors and singers and for a long time clergymen's sore throat has been recognized as an occupational risk of the Church.

Perhaps the best-known herb in this group is krameria (*Krameria triandra*), a small shrub that grows abundantly on the barren mountain slopes of Peru; hence its alternative name of Peruvian rhatany. At one time it was widely used in one of two forms: as a lozenge or pastille, sometimes combined with cocaine, and as a gargle. In a letter to the *Pharmaceutical Journal*, a pharmacist recently recalled memories of his early days as an apprentice in a pharmacy very near the Theatre Royal in Leeds, which:

> 'Had a large clientele of artistes who came not only for cosmetics and grease paints but also for advice and help in minor disasters such as a hangover and "relaxed throat".' For the latter the stock remedy was 'a gargle containing tincture of krameria and eau de cologne'. He adds: 'It certainly had a sound reputation among the Theatre Royal artistes.'

Older readers will recall, but may not associate with krameria, the wide publicity given in the 1930s to 'umckaloabo' (once nicely described as a 'substance which had nothing apart from its euphonious name to recommend it') in the treatment of tuberculosis. This, actually, was the swan-song of a story that went back to 1897 when a young Birmingham mechanic was found to have tuberculosis and, as was a common custom in those days, was advised to migrate to South Africa. This he did, where he met a local witch doctor who claimed to have a remedy, made from certain roots, for lung troubles. This he took for a couple of months, felt better, and returned to England where he was pronounced cured. At least he was fit enough to serve in the Boer War, attaining the rank of major. After the war he stayed on in South Africa and founded a company to market the herbal remedy that had 'cured' his tuberculosis, ultimately returning to London to push his product under the 'euphonious' name of 'umckaloabo'. This was the hey-day of quackery, and in 1909 the British Medical Association published a best-seller entitled *Secret Remedies: what they cost and what they contain*. According to this invaluable book umckaloabo contained alcohol, glycerin and krameria, and the ingredients of two and a half fluid ounces, sold at 5s a bottle, cost 1½d. Yet a quarter of a century later it was still able to hit the headlines.

Before coming to the final group of drugs to be considered in this category, a short note may be interpolated here, inspired by a comment that appeared in the *Pharmaceutical Journal*, the official journal of the Pharmaceutical Society of Great Britain, in the autumn of 1975 to the effect that 'it was somewhat perturbing to come across a report that a German drug manufacturer is taking an interest in that strange insectivore *Drosera rotundifolia*, and has offered to take as much as the Irish peat-lands can supply.' The *Journal*'s 'perturbation' was the perfectly laudable one that boglands possess a delicate ecological balance and are particularly vulnerable to depredations such as this.

The herbal interest is that this particular herb, also known as sundew and youthwort, has an old reputation as a remedy for chronic bronchitis, whooping-cough and asthma and their associated coughs. This is a reputation dating back to the days of Nicholas Culpeper who has been described as 'the doyen of herbal medicine in the first half of the seventeenth century'. It is interesting that it is still included in the official *Pharmacopoeias* of Austria, Belgium, France and Poland.

Like so many of these herbal remedies of old, it had a somewhat versatile reputation. Thus, it owes its name of sundew to the fact that in the seventeenth century the droplets on the leaf glands were used to remove sunburn and freckles. Youthwort as a name comes from the attribution described by Dr W T Fernie in *Herbal Simples*, published in 1895 as:

'Cattle of the female gender are said to have copulative instincts excited by eating even a small quantity of the plant (youthwort or lustwort).'

Be all that as it may, the interesting thing is that here is an old herbal remedy that has aroused sufficient interest in a modern pharmaceutical company to stimulate them to investigate its mode of action. Whether in due course it issues in a new modern format as a cough remedy, a cure for sunburn, or an aphrodisiac is beside the point. The relevant fact is that here would appear to be an example of what should be going on on a much larger scale in the way of modern research into the old claims for herbs that heal.

Finally there is a group of herbs that ease cough and its underlying cause by relaxing spasm of the bronchi or bronchioles (smaller bronchi). Bronchial spasm, of course, is the underlying cause of asthma, and here relief is obtained by more effective drugs, including ephedrine (see chapter 9) and adrenaline. In many cases of chronic bronchitis, however, there is an element of bronchial spasm, and in such patients a bronchodilator, as it is known, may be helpful. One useful herb in this context is lobelia (*Lobelia inflata*). It is also known as Indian tobacco, a name which it owes to the fact that it is indigenous to the eastern USA and has long been used by the Indians there as an expectorant. Early in the last century local doctors found it to be useful in asthma, and it was introduced to Britain for this purpose around 1830. There is another species indigenous to India.

Lobelia owes its bronchodilating action to an alkaloid, lobeline, which acquired a high reputation as a respiratory stimulant. For this purpose it was given by injection into the umbilical cords of new-born babies who were not breathing properly. It was also used as a stimulant of depressed breathing in adults, but has largely been replaced now by newer and more efficient drugs. It is still used, however, in cough mixtures for chronic bronchitis, as a constituent of asthma powders which are burnt and the smoke inhaled and, somewhat optimistically, in some anti-smoking pastilles. The rationale here is the interesting, and quite plausible, one that it has a nicotine-like action, and therefore if the cigarette addict takes it this will satisfy his craving for nicotine. Unfortunately, as so often happens, theory and practice have not coincided. On the other hand, this is yet another herb that scientific investigation has proved to have a justification for its use.

To conclude this chapter a much more recent example may be given of an old herbal remedy that has come into its own as a result of the laboratory. This is *Adhatoda vasica*, or Malabar nut, a shrub indigenous to India where it has long been used as an expectorant, as a reliever of cough and as a dilator of the bronchial tubes. In 1959 research workers in Baroda isolated from the leaves a new alkaloid which dilated the bronchi in experimental animals. Other workers confirmed this, and in due course a synthetic derivative of this active principle was put on the market under the name of bromhexine, which a report from the Department of Medicine in the University of Aberdeen has described as 'a valuable therapeutic advance in the difficult problem of aiding expectoration in the respiratory patient'.

The herbs reviewed in this chapter are a mixed bag. None of them may be curative, but all of them are herbs that heal. Between them they present an impressive case for the theme running through this book: that, while by no means in every case, yet in a not inconsiderable number of cases, the practice of our ancestors has been justified. As this is so, there is all the more reason why the research worker of today should be probing ever deeper into the healing mysteries of Nature.

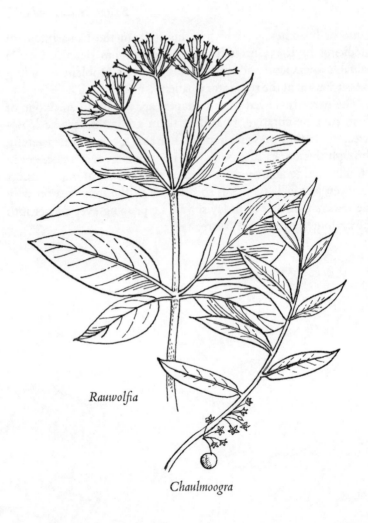

Rauwolfia

Chaulmoogra

9

The herbal wisdom
of the Orient

Traditionally, the Wise Men came from the East. This is one reason why the wise occidental should occasionally tear himself from his western treatises and research bench to cast an eye on what is happening in the Orient. Particularly is this true in the field of medicine which, with all respect to the many high-powered medical scientists in our midst, still refuses to fit itself into any narrow scientific classification. After all, the Chinese, for example, were practising an extraordinarily high standard of medicine and sanitation when their opposite numbers in the British Isles, for instance, were little more than barbarians.

Some two thousand years ago they produced an eighteen-volume textbook of medicine, entitled *Nei-ching*, which indicates that the Chinese of those days knew that the distribution of nutrition was one of the functions of the circulating blood, and this was followed by a textbook of treatment, *Shen Nung Ben Tsao*, which described the properties of more than 300 medicines. In 1578, Li Shih-chen, the great physician of the Ming dynasty, produced a book, entitled *Ben Ts'ao Kang Mu* (the *Chinese Pharmacopoeia*), which gave details of more than 1000 medical prescriptions, many of them still in use today. But still the search for herbs that heal continues, and within the last quarter of a century the Chinese have collected and identified another 2000 new medicinal herbs. Such is an indication of the medical riches of herbs, as yet strangely untouched by occidental science and medicine.

Not the least of the claims to fame of the Chinese is their adaptability, an interesting example of which was revealed in a paperback entitled *25 Years of Health Work*, published by the Democratic Republic of Vietnam in 1971. In this, much stress was laid on the extent to which the North Vietnamese had had to improvise medically during what was described as a quarter-century characterized by 'two devastating wars separated by a ten-year truce (1955–1964)'. This improvisation included making as full use as possible of traditional Chinese medicine and local drugs. Not only was the widespread cultivation of medicinal plants encouraged, but, it was claimed,

> 'It is usual for a peasant family to devote a patch of land to the cultivation of at least a dozen of the 58 so-called "family medicine" species, which provide for part of the family's needs while bringing in some extra income, as the State organizes the purchase of materia medica even from the remotest places.'

Here surely is do-it-yourself carried to a degree that even its most enthusiastic exponents in the West have not suggested. Indeed, there are still diehards in our midst who are reluctant to allow the sick citizen to prescribe for himself and his family. What would be their reaction or that of the Medicines Commission if the inflation-stricken British citizen were to revive the herb garden of old is anyone's guess. Latterly these gardens have tended to be more culinary than medicinal in content, but is there any reason why the modern gardener, or allotment holder, should not devote a corner of his garden, or allotment, to growing these 'excellent herbs' which, according to Kipling, 'our fathers had': 'excellent herbs to ease their pains'? After all, they could scarcely be more toxic than phenacetin, or even aspirin, of which our scientific pharmacologists are so fond.

This adaptability is not just a wartime measure, but a matter of national policy. This is admirably brought out in *Chinese Medicine As We Saw It*, a publication of the John Fogarty International Center for Advanced Study in Health Services, published in 1974 by the US Department of Health, Education, and Welfare. It consists of a series of reports by 'distinguished medical visitors', mainly citizens of the USA who have recently visited the People's Republic of China. Each contributor stresses how consistent current Chinese medical thinking is that the best progress can be made by a mingling of western medicine and the traditional medicine of China. The emphasis is on the latter, but, if it is not adequate for treating a given patient, then there are no scruples or hesitation about calling in the aid of western medicine.

This approach is highlighted in the field of treatment where, as one contributor puts it:

> 'Throughout China a very high priority has been awarded research efforts into the medical use of herbs. Teams of experts, using pharmaceutical assay equipment, are conducting exhaustive tests in the search for new and better remedies.' 'Although', he adds, 'some researchers are seeking specific answers to explain the curative qualities of certain plant substances, most, which have survived the test of centuries, are being left alone.'

At the Tientsin Herbal Institute, a research institute on traditional drugs founded towards the end of the 1950s, employing 153 people, and one of fifty similar research establishments, he found that a hundred different herbs were being currently assayed for anti-cancer properties. This has a high priority in China, along with research into the treatment of heart disease and chronic bronchitis.

Other drugs he found that were being investigated were *Iris palosii* for a contraceptive agent, a derivative of soya bean for psoriasis, and an alkaloid isolated from a plant named *Anisodus tanguticus* which was claimed to have proved useful in the treatment of toxic shock. Also interesting was 'a unique form of acupuncture', in which this traditional method of treatment was accompanied by the injection of medicinal herbs.

The report dealing with heart disease states that in a traditional hospital in Shanghai successful results were being obtained from the use of 'an old herbal medicine', *Salvia miltiorrhiza*, to relieve the pain of coronary thrombosis. Much attention is being devoted to the problem of schistosomiasis, the most important parasitic disease in China – as in many other parts of Asia and Africa. Not much progress is being made in the treatment of the disease, though pumpkin seeds are proving useful as an ancillary to other drugs, and the root of the wild lily (*Hemerocallis thunbergii*) has been found effective, but unpleasantly toxic, in clinical trials. More success is being achieved in the search for preparations that will kill the snails that transmit the disease to man. The most promising is the fruit residue of the tea plant, *Thea oleosa*, but unfortunately, it is proving toxic to fish, a very definite drawback from the practical point of view. There is little point in saving the populace from schistosomiasis, only to allow them to die from inanition as a result of being deprived of a staple source of food. A range of other plants or herbs, including the rose tree (*Rhododendron sinensis*), spurge, aconite, poison oak and raspberry, have proved promising initially in this respect and are undergoing further investigation.

The ramifications of schistosomiasis as one of the major health problems of Asia and Africa justifies a sudden leap at this stage to Abyssinia, where, while engaged on a survey of the disease, Dr

Akluku Lemma of Haile Selassie University, Addis Ababa, happened to notice on one of his trips into Northern Ethiopia a large collection of dead snails downstream from a village washing place. What intrigued him was that upstream and farther downstream the snails were abundant and thriving. This state of affairs he tracked down to the fact that the 'soap' the village women used for washing their clothes was made from the ground berries of the endod bush. On investigation these berries were found to be fatal to snails (or molluscicidal, to use the technical term) as well as having soap-like, or detergent, properties. Not only are these berries effective in killing snails, doing so in a dilution of 15 to 30 parts per million, but they are harmless to mammals and other plants, and the endod bush (*Phytolacca dodecandra*) is popular as a hedge in the villages of northern Ethiopia.

Here then seemed to be the ideal answer to schistosomiasis, which is endemic in Ethiopia – at least in this region. If the local snails could be killed, the causal parasite (*Schistosoma haematobium*) could not be transmitted to the local population and therefore the infestation would for all practical purposes disappear, or at least be radically reduced. Further, the fact that the endod berries were harmless to animals and other plants meant that they could be used without any fear of the local inhabitants being freed from schistosomiasis, only to die of starvation because the cattle, fish and crops were being killed by the molluscicide. In addition, the fact that the endod bush grew so freely meant that the snail-killer could be cheaply produced. And so it turned out to be. The berries were bought in the local market, ground in the mills used by the villagers to grind their chili peppers, and then applied along the banks of the local streams in watering cans every month or couple of months – with a most gratifying drop in the incidence of the disease. The Chinese may not yet have been as lucky as the Ethiopians, but it is certainly not for want of trying, and there can be little doubt that one day, and probably sooner rather than later, they will successfully rid their teeming millions of this hazard to life and health.

Where the Chinese do seem to have scored, however, in a somewhat similarly accidental manner, is in the chance discovery of the possible medical application of what are known as the gibberellins. These are a group of naturally occurring plant hormones of complex chemical structure that have been isolated from plant materials, and in particular from immature bean seeds. Their main source, however, is the fungus, *Gibberella fujikuroi*. This fungus first achieved fame, or rather notoriety, during the last century as a serious blight of rice. In the course of investigating this the Japanese discovered that sterile filtrates from the fungus stimulated the growth of rice rather than nullified it, and in due course a pure crystalline substance was isolated and given the name of gibberellin. This, acting as a growth hormone, is now used on a wide scale for stimulating, not only the growth of rice – and thus converting a blight into a boon – but also many other plants as well.

An old Chinese lady decided to try it out on her troublesome ulcerated legs, presumably on the principle that if it was good for rice and made it nice and healthy, it would have the same effect on her ulcerated legs, and she was right. After a few applications the ulcerated skin finally healed. Like all such natural unorthodox cures this aroused widespread local interest and, being modern China, this was soon translated into action. Here was a cure in the best tradition of Chinese medicine. A clinical trial was launched in several hospitals, including a People's Liberation Army Hospital, and within eight months over a thousand patients with various skin diseases had been successfully treated. And if it could cure ulcerated skin, why not ulcers elsewhere? The answer to which is, in the words of the USA report, that:

'Preliminary findings suggest that "920" [the "trade name"

for gibberellins in China] is effective in treating other types of diseases, including ulcerations of the stomach and duodenum.'

One herb not mentioned in the USA report, which is well known in China, is one species of fritillary which has a reputation for the treatment of cancer of the breast and for increasing lactation.

But the best known of all proven drugs that have come out of China is the one we know as ephedrine, which comes from a Chinese herb that has been used medicinally in China for more that four millenniums. Ma Huang, as it is known in China, is derived from several species of *Ephedra*, two of which are indigenous to China, one to India and one to India and Spain. Ephedrine has had a slow transition to western medicine. In spite of the long history of Ma Huang in China, it was only in 1887 that ephedrine was isolated from it, and it was practically half a century later before the full medicinal value of ephedrine was realized as a most useful reliever of asthma and other allergic conditions, that could be taken by mouth. Hitherto such patients had had to have injections of adrenaline to get the requisite relief. Now, however, in all except acute cases, they could get relief without the necessity of an injection.

The Chinese drug, however, that today is arousing most interest in the West is ginseng. Esteemed, indeed honoured, in China for somewhere in the region of 4000 years, it has slowly percolated west through the Far East and Russia to the pharmacological laboratories of the West, until in 1975 it was included in the programme of a five-day international symposium in Switzerland, in which the World Health Organization participated. It is official in the *Japanese Pharmacopoeia* and *Russian Pharmacopoeia*. Yet ask a random dozen British doctors what they know about it, and the chances are that the only response will be blank stare. This is scarcely surprising when it is realized that in *Martindale*, the doctors' therapeutic *vade-mecum*, it is only referred to in small type in one of the terminal sections entitled 'Supplementary Drugs and Ancillary Substances', with the laconic comment:

'Ginseng has demulcent properties and is reputed to have a sedative effect on the cerebrum and a mildly stimulating action on the vital centres. It has been given in fatigue, hypotonia and neurasthenia.'

Yet this is not a case of deliberately damning with faint praise. Paradoxically, it is a fair summing up of the available scientific evidence. The paradox is that so many of the impartial experts who have considered the pros and cons of the plant, in spite of the lack of any really hard scientific facts to bite on, end up by making what can best be described as encouraging noises. Two such British experts, both held in high esteem in that branch of the study of drugs known as pharmacognosy (the scientific study of naturally occurring substances with a medicinal action), may be quoted. One, writing in 1973, said that recent work had shown quite clearly that:

'The ginseng root contains saponin glycosides ... which are mainly responsible for its stimulant effect and for in-creasing non-specific resistance against harmful external agencies of a physical, chemical, and biological kind.' According to the other, writing two years later: 'There seems little doubt that ginseng and its relatives have a con-tribution to make in medicine but the value of this contri-bution depends largely on satisfactory clinical evaluation, adequate supplies of raw materials and an intelligent use of these materials.'

The hard facts about ginseng can be briefly summarized. It is the dried root of two species of *Panax*: *Panax ginseng* (or *Panax schinseng* as it is sometimes known) and *Panax quinquefolium*. The former is the original source and is still considered the best, and grows wild in north-eastern Asia. For a long time the wild form, particularly that from Manchuria, was considered the best, but cultivation has become necessary to meet the demand, and this is done in China, Russia and Northern Korea for these countries. The demand from other parts of the world is met by cultivation in Southern Korea, Japan and Canada. *Panax quinquefolium* is the species that grows wild in Canada and the eastern USA. The generic name, *Panax*, has the same derivation as panacea – or 'all-heal', while the Chinese name Jin-chen, means 'manlike', and is derived from the fact that the roots vaguely resemble the arms, body and legs of a human doll. According to the doctrine of signatures therefore this is a plant that will heal all ailments in any part of the body.

And such was, and is, its reputation: the ultimate elixir of life, a symbol of strength and long life, the source of happiness, a tonic and an aphrodisiac. Mention your desire in life, and ginseng will satisfy it. In more prosaic terms it was also recommended for anaemia, diabetes, insomnia and neurasthenia – all conditions, it will be noted, characterized by exhaustion and a lack of zest for life. The difficulty is to convert this into the more precise concrete terms of modern medicine.

Part of the trouble may lie in the complex biochemical structure of the root, which may explain some of the contradictory reports that have appeared. Thus Japanese research workers have recently isolated five active principles from it, and shown that these stimulate what has been described as 'every conceivable aspect' of protein metabolism. This fits in with the hitherto suspiciously vague claims of its action, and we must now await with what patience we possess until further work can be carried out with these purified active principles, which should throw light on what precisely this ancient herbal remedy can do – as well as how it does it.

The work done on experimental animals suggests that it improves the running and swimming ability of rats and protects animals from some of the effects of physical stress such as exposure to heat or cold, prolonged immobilization, low atmospheric pressures and infection with various micro-organisms. Comparable results have been reported in man. One Bulgarian research worker who has been studying the plant for over twenty years reports that:

> 'Ginseng should not be regarded merely as a non-specific stimulant of the excitation process but also as a pharmacological agent which improves the responses of tissue structures. In many persons – but not all – it delays mental and physical fatigue.'

Which is presumably why it is regularly given to Russian cosmonauts on space missions.

From all this it is difficult to draw anything like precise conclusions. It is easy to be sceptical but, as one American writer has put it: 'One can't help wondering how any absolutely inert substance could for ages, and in widely separated lands, maintain so high a reputation.' The 'mysterious East' still shrouds this millennium-old herb in its veil, but it looks as if the time were coming when the down-to-earth Occident was about to get down to the task of probing the mystery. After all, if we can probe the mysteries of outer space, surely we can find out whether or not this ancient Chinese drug does what its protagonists claim it has done for the last four thousand years and more.

All in all, Chinese medicine has much to offer us in the way of 'herbs that heal'. As Dr James Y P Chen states in *Medicine and Public Health in the People's Republic of China*, another of the excellent publications of the Fogarty International Center:

> 'The Chinese materia medica is a vast storehouse of complex, loosely structured, pharmacological information subject to

scientific screening and verification. In the past, western medicine has gained immeasurably from chance discovery and application of ancient oriental medicinals. Ephedrine (*Ma Huang* from China) and *Rauwolfia serpentina* (from India) are two classic examples of the application of western science and technology to traditional herbal remedies. It is conceivable other herbal medicaments with equal potential to western scientific and medical areas of interest exist. Such areas of interest may well include the treatment of cancer, viral disease, leukaemia, and perhaps neuromuscular ailments such as muscular dystrophy and poliomyelitis. A key programme launched by western scientific and medical professions to conduct an investigation into Chinese medical practices and medicines would be fraught with frustration and difficulties, but the pay-off may well be worth the effort.'

Indian civilization is one of the oldest on earth and, like the Chinese, it has made many contributions to advances in medicine. Among the many healing herbs we owe to India are opium, aconite, acacia, cinnamon, ginger, chenopodium and chaulmoogra. Of all these perhaps the most intriguing is chaulmoogra, or hydnocarpus, oil, until a couple of decades ago the only drug of any value in the treatment of leprosy. As Dr Robert Cochrane, the outstanding leprologist of his time, commented in 1964:

'When we review the long history of leprosy, one outstanding drug, which has until recently always been in the forefront is chaulmoogra (hydnocarpus) oil and its derivatives. This remedy held pride of place in the treatment of leprosy for centuries and was the basis of all specific therapy in leprosy until it was largely discarded when sulphones were introduced.'

First introduced to orthodox medicine for the treatment of leprosy by a British surgeon of the Indian Medical Service in 1854, it had for long been a well-known indigenous remedy for leprosy. Tradition has it that it is a form of treatment based on ancient Burmese folklore. The rather delightful story of its introduction for this purpose is that a Burmese prince discovered he had leprosy and was directed by the gods to withdraw from the world and meditate in the depths of the forest. He dutifully did this and in due course was directed to a tree with a large fruit in which there were many seeds which he was told to eat. As a result of this his leprosy was cured.

Of the 1800 species of plants with medicinal or toxic properties which, according to the Indian Council of Scientific and Industrial Research, are known to grow in India (and this is a minimum figure), undoubtedly the best known is *Rauwolfia serpentina*. In the 1950s it leapt into fame as, at that time, a new entity in the drug world – a tranquillizer: a therapeutic genus which, plugged in a big way by the pharmaceutical industry, sold by it through complaisant doctors to the long-suffering public, threatened to lull Western civilization into a state of mental and emotional apathy from which we are still suffering. So excited did the pharmaceutical industry become about it, particularly in the USA, that they practically cleared every single plant out of India, and thereby forced the Indian Government to ban its export. This is an example of disgraceful exploitation which, unfortunately, is not unique in the industry's annals. Granted that it was also proving to be a most effective plant for bringing high blood pressure under control but, as the Scottish minister is said to have exclaimed when his prayer for rain after a long drought was suddenly drowned by a torrential downpour rattling on the corrugated roof of his church, 'Oh Lord we thank Thee, but, Oh Lord, do show some sense of discrimination.'

Beyond this sudden leap to fame – and notoriety – lies its

history stretching back several thousand years as a soother of the mind and an antidote to lunacy. It had become incorporated into the folklore of India to such an extent that it was regularly chewed by the holy men of the country seeking tranquillity for their meditations, and Gandhi is said to have been a regular drinker of a tea made from it. The root, popularly known as 'snake-root' because of its long, tapering, crooked nature, contains most of the medicinal properties of the plant, which covers the foothills of certain parts of India, where it is gathered by the natives who pound it into a powder before using it. It is to its snake-like character that it owes its species name of *serpentina*, and, on the principle of the doctrine of signatures, this also dictated that it should be used for the treatment of snake bite. Its genus name was given to it in the sixteenth century in honour of Leonard Rauwolf, one of the best-known physician-botanists of that time.

Gradually over the years it became a common prescription for all sorts of mental diseases and when, in the post-1918 era Indian chemists began to analyse it and isolate its active principles, these were even more widely used for their characteristic tranquillizing, relaxing and calming effects. In due course Indian doctors working with mental patients began to notice that rauwolfia often produced a lowering of the blood pressure, and by the 1940s, it has been estimated, at least a million Indians were receiving preparations of rauwolfia for high blood pressure. Yet still the Occident was not interested.

Then, in 1949, an article appeared in the *British Heart Journal* in which Dr Rustom Jal Vakil, the distinguished Indian cardiologist, reported that he had had satisfactory experience with the drug for ten years, and that forty-six out of fifty Indian physicians, whom he had consulted by post, were in favour of it, compared with all others, for the treatment of high blood pressure. In an account of his own experience of the drug he reported that 44% of his patients with high blood pressure showed a definite lowering of it when given rauwolfia. This report was read, inwardly digested and acted on by Dr Robert W Wilkins, Chief of the Hypertension Clinic of the Massachusetts General Hospital, Boston – with correspondingly satisfactory results. Typical of his findings are the following conclusions.

'These clinical experiences with rauwolfia preparations have taught us that they are more than just further additions to the rapidly growing list of hypotensive agents ... Current indications are that these preparations may find their chief usefulness in many psychoneuroses and tension states, in addition to essential hypertension ... Its most beneficial effect is to decrease "neurotic" symptoms in all patients and to lower the blood pressure, particularly in young, labile hypertensive subjects with tachycardia.'

This unleashed the flood-gates of the pharmaceutical industry, whose scouts started scouring the earth for rauwolfia. This, they soon found, was fairly widely scattered through the tropics with the exception of Australia, but the two most potent sources of the active principles were *Rauwolfia serpentina* in Burma, Thailand and Java, and *Rauwolfia vomitoria*, or African rauwolfia, which is indigenous to tropical Africa from the Guinea coast to Mozambique. In the course of time the main constituent, reserpine, was synthesized, but much of it still comes from the dried roots of either *R. serpentina* or *R. vomitoria*.

After hitting the headlines and becoming a best-seller both for the treatment of high blood pressure and as a tranquillizer, rauwolfia is now slightly under a cloud, for a variety of reasons. One is the inevitable reaction to the over-enthusiastic claims made for it originally by both the pharmaceutical industry and doctors. Another is the equally inevitable, if unfortunate, fact about the pharmaceutical industry that it must always be stimulating sales: one of the best ways to do this, whether you are selling drugs, motor cars, or detergents, is to produce a new product. Another reason is the production of new hypotensive, or blood-pressure lowering, agents that are more effective. Finally there is a reason that is beginning to worry not a few experts in this field.

This arises out of the fundamentally sound reasoning that when investigating the activity of a new drug, one of the first things to do is to isolate the active principle or principles. As often as not this results in the separation out of a multiplicity of such principles as, for example, in the case of the foxglove, ergot, and the poppy. Occasionally, as in the case of *ephedra*, there is only one, ephedrine, of any value. In the case of the producers of multiple principles, there may be ultimate confusion; again, as in the case of the fox-glove and ergot, the manufacturers, with their research workers, become too clever and decide that one principle, either natural or synthesized, is all that is required. Particularly is this the case if the principle can be easily synthesized, because every chemical company prefers the straightforward laboratory synthesis of a drug to the messy procedure of isolating it from a plant.

In practice, however, this does not always work out and, often for unknown reasons, the isolated principle is not as effective as the whole plant, or it may be as effective but more toxic. This is a problem that has already been highlighted in chapter 2 on herbs and the heart, and it is one that is being discussed in the case of rauwolfia. Is it possible that an extract of the root, containing its active principles, or alkaloids, is more effective and safer than the isolated principles? Is it not possible that there is some reason for there being such a multiplicity of alkaloids in any given plant, and that the combination is therefore the best way to use the plant, even though its action in certain respects may not be as potent as that of the individual constituents? And after all, as we are learning to our cost, safety is as important in drugs as efficiency. Alternatively, is there not a risk that in purifying and repurifying a plant extract when searching for its active principles in glorious isolation, the therapeutic potency may be lost? Certainly this is a hazard that is worrying some of the more responsible research workers investigating ginseng. It is an old, old story that it is easy to be too clever and, as often as not, there is no one more blinkered in this way than the pharmacologist, whether he be academic or industrial.

Be all that as it may, however, rauwolfia is an outstanding contribution to the list of herbs that heal, and one of which India has every reason to be proud. It may be under a cloud in the Occident at the moment, but it is by no means dead. Indeed, it has only just surfaced in an entirely new role – for treating frostbite.

As a footnote or appendage it may not be remiss to be reminded that rauwolfia is proving of value in the veterinary field. The ageing male turkey is liable to develop high blood pressure, and this may prove fatal by rupturing his aorta, which is the artery leading from the heart to the circulatory system. Whether this be the price he pays for his outbursts of temper is an open question but, whatever the cause, it can result in quite serious economic loss. An enterprising American veterinary surgeon therefore had the bright idea at the height of rauwolfia's two-pronged reputation as a hypotensive drug and a tranquillizer, of trying it out on turkeys by adding it to their drinking water: it worked. At least, it lowered their blood pressure and thus preserved their lives which was the main thing, though, alas, it did not apparently moderate their outbursts of wild rage.

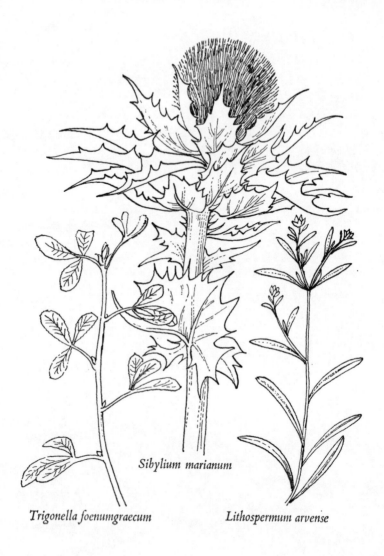

Sibylium marianum

Trigonella foenumgraecum

Lithospermum arvense

10
Fertility and infertility

Dr Hastings Kamuzu Banda, President of Malawi, was given his second name, which means 'a little root', to commemorate the ending of his mother's barrenness by a potion prepared from herbs by a medicine man. He was the first child of the marriage. Whether *propter hoc* or merely *post hoc* may be arguable, it is an episode symptomatic of the tremendous faith that mankind has always had in the power of herbs to control fertility. All down the ages herbs, with or without incantations, astrology, and magical or religious rites, have been used as aphrodisiacs, abortifacients and contraceptives. Indeed, there are few herbs that have not been used for one or other of these purposes at some time or another since Adam and Eve were expelled from the Garden of Eden.

As the propagation of the race is one of the primeval instincts, this search for fertility is scarcely surprising. What is rather more surprising is the age-old search for contraceptives, a reminder that birth control dates back long before the days of Marie Stopes in the United Kingdom and Margaret Sanger in the USA. Indeed, the bright young things of today might well be able to learn quite a lot from what their forebears knew about sex.

To the anthropologist, one of the many intriguing problems

is how primitive tribes did, and do, manage to delay first pregnancies. There is a popular belief that in the 'good old days' before the Welfare State was invented, large families were the rule, for the very sound reason that an ample supply of sons was the best insurance for old age. This may have been the case in certain civilizations at certain periods of time, but it was by no means universal. Abortion may have been a common method of coping with the problem, whether marital, premarital or extramarital, partly because it was relatively easier to find a herb that would induce abortion than one that would prevent conception. It must have been evident to 'interested parties' at a fairly early stage of human development that a strong purgative, for example, was liable to be accompanied by the expulsion of any conceptus that might be present. Hence the large number of herbs with purgative action, such as aloes, that were also used as abortifacients. It is a tradition that still persists, and in the pre-'pill' days a certain proprietary preparation, 'worth a guinea a box', enjoyed a wide popularity among certain social classes as a useful guarantee against unwanted pregnancy.

The problems of infertility and contraception are more complex and correspondingly more fascinating. Here magical and psychological factors play a larger part. Fear may induce abortion – though, in parenthesis, a factor too often overlooked is that it can be extraordinarily difficult to persuade a healthy uterus to part with its contents except by physical means – but it is much more likely to interfere with conception. Hence the importance of psychological factors in coping with the infertile couple, and the difficulty in deciding whether in such cases subsequent fertility is the result of the herb (or drug) being given or psychological factors such as faith in the doctor, or witch doctor. The same difficulty arises in assessing the value of any drug or herb in this sphere where apparently successful contraception may actually be the result of infertility.

Two herbal contraceptives of folklore that have undergone careful examination are species of the genus *Lithospermum*. One of these, *Lithospermum ruderale*, also known as gromwell and stone-seed, and indigenous to the western side of the USA, is used as an oral contraceptive by the Soshon Indians of Nevada. The other, *Lithospermum arvense*, is used for the same purpose in Central Europe. In both cases the evidence is reasonably well authenticated, and experimental investigations have shown that an extract of *L. ruderale*, and of another species, *L. officinalis* (the leaves of which, incidentally, are used to make Bohemian or Croatian tea) suppress oestrus in rats and mice. In passing it is worthy of note that these investigations brought out a point that crops up again and again in considering herbal remedies. This is that the potency of different extracts of the plant supplied for investigation varied considerably: this variability was confirmed in the course of this investigation in preparing the various extracts from *L. officinale*, when it was found that slow drying seemed to destroy activity, whereas quick drying did not.

The real significance of these findings, however, so far as contraception is concerned, is that they indicate that *Lithospermum* owes its contraceptive reputation in North America and Central Europe to its ability to interfere with oestrous, or ovulation, and, as every woman knows, this is how the 'pill' acts. It is a hormone mixture that interferes with ovulation and thereby prevents sperm meeting ovum – with all the resulting consequences. This may well also be the *modus operandi* of herbal contraceptives and, as. will be discussed shortly, it has evoked a search in the plant world for plants with hormone-like activities. *Lithospermum* is one genus that falls into this category, and several of its sixty species have been found to have hormonal activity.

Another plant in this category is the garden pea (*Pisum sativum*), one of the oldest foods of mankind. It has been cultivated from ancient times, judging from the finding of fossil remains of it in Swiss lake villages. On the other hand, it never seems to have had a medicinal reputation, and it only aroused medical interest some thirty years ago when loss of fertility in rats was attributed to it. The resulting pharmacological investigation indicated that an oil extracted from it reduced fertility in rats, attributed at first to an anti-vitamin effect, but finally associated with interference with the hormonal cycle of ovulation. In due course the intriguing suggestion was thrown out that the reduced fertility of Tibetans was due to peas being one of their staple articles of diet; claims were also made that this contraceptive action of an oil from garden peas had been confirmed in clinical trials. These results are still awaiting confirmation.

Even more intriguing in this context is the family of plants known as Verbenaceae, which consists of 200 genera and 2600 species, some of which have hormonal activity. These include vervain, the only species native to Britain. With a reputation as a sacred or magic herb dating back to the days of ancient Persia, its multiplicity of names displays its versatility. Included among these is the herb of the Cross because of the story that it was found on Calvary and used to help to staunch the bleeding from wounds of the crucified Christ: today it is still called herbe sacrée in France. To the Romans it was herba sacra or herba veneris as it was dedicated to Venus in their altar worship, while to the Welsh in the Middle Ages it was devil's bane: after cutting it in the darkness of night it was taken into their churches to use as a sprinkler of holy water. Coming down to earth with a bump, it was known in Britain as pigeon's meat, for the simple reason that pigeons like it.

Against this allegorical background it had an equally versatile medicinal reputation, dating back to Hippocrates, when it was used as an antidote to plague and the ague. Indeed, it is said that until quite recently – and for all I know it may still be the custom – in some rural areas the root was tied round the neck with a ribbon as protection against ague, or rheumatics. Among the many other complaints it cured were migraine, insomnia, asthma, inflamed eyes and sore throats. It also stood in high repute as a hair tonic. Needless to say, its dedication to Venus indicates its aphrodisiac properties but, though it is now known to contain a hormone-like substance, there seems to be no reference to its use as a contraceptive.

On the other hand, however, and illustrating the perpetual difficulty in sifting the evidence presented by the history and reputation of many of these old herbal remedies, there is another drug derived from this family of verbenaceae, whose name, *Agnus Castus*, is derived from its Mediterranean source of origin, *Vitex agnus-castus*, the 'chaste tree'. Of this a seventeenth century apothecary is recorded as saying:

> 'It cohibits the motion of sperm, and allays venerous fancies in the night, for which cause the Athenian matrons in their Feasts to Ceres, the better to custodite their chastity, strewed their bed with its leafs.'

The fruits, too, seemed to have an anti-aphrodisiac action and were at one time official in the *Spanish Pharmacopoeia*. Its contents resemble those of vervain. It is difficult to distinguish truth and legend in this pleasingly mixed story, but on general principles the finding of a hormone-like constituent suggests that the anti-aphrodisiac reputation of the fruits internally, if not of the leaves externally, is the more likely. On the other hand, it could be argued that it was as a contraceptive that it commended itself to the devotees of Venus.

Before passing to the culmination of this tale of how herbs are making one of the greatest contributions to the future welfare of mankind, two other popular herbal remedies may be mentioned, not because of any proof of their having hormone constituents, but because of the temptation to suggest such a possibility. One is motherwort, or *Leonurus cardiaca*, which owes its popular name to the fact that, according to Nicholas Culpeper, in *The Complete Herbal* (1653), 'it makes women joyful mothers of children, and settles their wombs as they may, therefore we call it Motherwort'. This is translated into more prosaic language by another writer who states that it is used for 'female hysteria, to control menstruation and tone the membranes of the uterus, and as an aphrodisiac'. The other is milk thistle, or *Sibylium marianum*, declared by John Evelyn to be 'a great breeder of milk and a proper diet for wet nurses'. Its popular name, as well as another of its names, Virgin's milk, are linked with the legend that the characteristic white veins on its leaves were made by the Virgin Mary's milk as she fed the Holy Child. Whatever the significance of these popular reputations, is it possible that there may be a more prosaic explanation: that both herbs have a hormone-like activity associated with both pregnancy and lactation?

The current era, when the world is largely dependent upon herbs for its oral contraceptives and for many of the important hormones necessary for the treatment of the ills to which women are heir, began in 1949 when the workers at the Mayo Clinic announced to the world the quite dramatic effects produced by cortisone in alleviating rheumatoid arthritis. Unfortunately, the only known source of cortisone was desoxycholic acid from ox bile and, if the claims for cortisone were confirmed, then more than ten times the entire cattle population of the USA would be necessary to provide cortisone for the arthritics of the republic. Further, the process of manufacture was a complicated thirty-two stage procedure, as expensive as it was complex.

The obvious alternative source was the group of steroidal saponins, as they are known, found in certain plants, and chemically related to cortisone. The most likely plant source was *Strophanthus*, and in due course, though by no means speedily, a botanical expedition was sent to tropical Africa to find out whether any species of *Strophanthus* produced sufficient of these sapogenins to justify their collection for the commercial production of cortisone. The expedition was a failure from this point of view, though much valuable botanical information was acquired; and more than one member of the party came back a sadder, but wiser, man with an increased respect for Nature and the plant world.

Perhaps the fundamental lesson learned was one that was already known to, or at least suspected by, really experienced botanists. This was that, not only can the amount of a given substance vary from species to species of a given genus, it can also vary tremendously (from nil to large amounts) in the same species from different geographical locations. Thus, in the search for the sapogenin, sarmentogenin, as a precursor of cortisone, twenty species of *Strophanthus*, and twenty-three samples of one species, *Strophanthus sarmentosus*, were collected in the course of a 16,000-mile trek through a dozen countries in tropical Africa, but not one of them contained the desired compound. This was no isolated experience. Professor T Reichstein, of Basle, who shared the Nobel Prize in 1950 with Professor Kendall, the Mayo Clinic biochemist, and Dr Philip Hench, the Mayo Clinic rheumatologist, examined fifty different African species of *Strophanthus* but found appreciable amounts of sarmentogenin in only one of them.

It was a salutary lesson, with much wider implications than had previously been recognized. For, not only does the content of a herb or plant vary from species to species and from area to area, it can also vary according to the time of day and the time of year: a point which has already been fully discussed in chapter 1.

Fortunately, the failure of *Strophanthus* as a precursor of cortisone – and in due course of sex hormones – was not a serious matter, partly because methods of manufacturing cortisone became simpler, and therefore cheaper, partly because other sources of precursors were found among the yams, or *Dioscoreae*, of Mexico. For a long time, tubers of many of the yams have been used for food as they are rich in starch and today, not only those of Mexico, but many of the other 600 species are among the most valuable plants we possess. In fact they are largely responsible for the fact that plants are today the most important source of raw material for the world's steroid industry. Thus, of the 1000 tons of raw steroid used in 1973, 77% came from plant sources (50% from Mexico, 15% from the USA, 6% from Africa, 5% from China and 1% from India), 10% from animal sources, and the remainder from total synthesis. Around one quarter of this grand total was used in making the 'pill'.

Some idea of what is involved in this commercial exploitation of the yam to prevent human beings from multiplying too freely can be obtained from the fact that, because cultivation is uneconomic, collection has to be from the yam in the wild, and this is done principally in Mexico, Guatemala, India, Tibet and China. In order to acquire the 56% of raw steroid (in the form of diosgenin, the sapogenin present in yams) used in 1973, 112,000 tons of fresh tuber, with a moisture content of 90%, had to be collected.

While yams are the main source of precursors of sex hormones, several cultivated plants are also being exploited for this purpose. One of these is fenugreek seed (*Trigonella foenumgraecum*), an annual herb indigenous to the eastern Mediterranean, and cultivated in Egypt, Morocco and India. It was well known to the ancients, being one of the constituents of the embalming and incense oil used by the Egyptians. Its most interesting medicinal reputation is as a stimulant of lactation and for the 'encouragement of an alluring roundness of the breast', for which purpose it was – and still may be – used by the ladies of the harems of North Africa and the Middle East. The intriguing question arises as to whether there is any association between the reputed action on the breast and its current reputation as a source or a precursor of the sex hormones. On a more plebeian level it was widely used as a demulcent to soothe chapped hands and lips and disordered digestive tracts. Otherwise, until its discovery as a source of diosgenin, its only claim to fame was as a spice in curry and in veterinary practice.

Another source is various species of *Agave*, of which there are 300. The most useful from the point of view of precursors of sex hormones is *Agave sisalana*, or sisal. Here the precursor is obtained from the leaf waste stripped from the leaves during removal of the fibre. The juice from this waste is allowed to ferment for seven days and then provides a most useful source of another sapogenin, hecogenin which is converted into sex hormones in Britain and Italy, and provides a most helpful addition to the income of East Africa. It can also be obtained from one of the species in tropical America, *Agave americana*.

A third source is cultivated soya bean, from which yet another sapogenin, stigmasterol, is obtained in the USA. Soya, or soy, bean (*Glycine soja*) has been cultivated in China for practically five thousand years. Although it was introduced to Europe in the seventeenth century and North America at the beginning of the nineteenth century, it was not until after the turn of the present century that it was commercially exploited outside China. Now, of the thirty million tons of beans produced annually, just under 60% come from China and 35% from the USA. Hitherto regarded as a rich source of fats and proteins essential to the survival of the human race (as discussed in chapter 11) it is now subserving this further useful function in helping to keep down the number of hungry mouths that have to be fed.

Such then is the contribution of herbs to some of the many problems presented to the human race by its potent instinct for reproduction, whether curbing it or stimulating it. It may not be a process of healing in the strict, or personal, sense of the term, but from the point of view of human happiness it is one of the most helpful roles herbs can play. Once the exaggerations of the current women's liberation movement sink into the past, and men and women realize and accept that the two prime functions of the sexual impulse are reproduction and mutual understanding, and that never the twain should part if true happiness is to be achieved, then the age-old reputation of herbs in this field will come to fulfilment.

Meanwhile much still remains to be done in the way of investigating more herbs that have a traditional reputation either for controlling or stimulating the sexual impulse, or for producing abortion when this is called for. We must not repeat the frequent mistake of doctors and the pharmaceutical industry of becoming obsessed with a one-track mind. The current exploitation of herbs as a precursor of the sex hormones is all to the good, but already people should be quietly following up other herbal approaches to the subject. Almost certainly Nature has as many new secrets to reveal to us in this area in the future, as she has revealed to us in the past.

Among these, it is hoped, is an alternative, safer 'pill' based on some other rationale than that of interfering with the hormonal balance of women throughout their childbearing span of life. That it is as safe as it has proved to be so far is something to be thankful for, but what is too often forgotten is that to be effective it has to be taken for a period of some thirty years. What we do not yet know therefore is its ultimate long-term effect. The risk of its increasing the incidence of cancer after the menopause may be doubtful but cannot altogether be ruled out and, though one is prepared to take risks with drugs when dealing with illness or disease, we are here dealing with healthy members of the community. To expose them to unnecessary hazards to life and health is a responsibility that at times our administrators and their statistical advisers are accepting in too facile a manner.

As Professor Victor Wynn, Professor of Human Metabolism at St Mary's Hospital, London, has commented:

'We keep saying how safe it is and how much research has been done, but there has never been a deep penetrating analysis of all the metabolic effects. There is still a great deal to be learnt, and it will be learnt only if there is a willingness of all sides to do research. There must be less complacency.'

Even on a shorter-term point of view, there is a worrying accumulation of disturbing evidence. Thus, 1975 saw the publication in Britain of a book entitled *Neurological Complications of Oral Contraceptives*. The mere fact that a reputable publisher felt it to be worth while publishing such a book is in itself evidence of a state of affairs that cannot be regarded with complacency, a reaction supported by the comments of one medical reviewer when he said: 'The commoner cerebrovascular episodes are discussed fully; the much rarer conditions, such as chorea, polyneuropathy, and myasthenic states, are also mentioned.' Masterly understatement may be a traditional trade-mark of the Englishman, but to refer in this casual manner to strokes and the like being 'the commoner' complications of a medicament given so freely to healthy women is somewhat worrying.

Equally unsettling is an annotation which appeared in *The Lancet* in 1975, entitled 'Oral Contraceptives and Liver Tumours', and based on a monograph published by the International Agency for Cancer Research. The gist of this is that thirteen months before the group responsible for the monograph first met, there appeared the first of several reports (nineteen cases in *The Lancet* and the *British Medical Journal*) of liver tumours in women taking oral contraceptives. These tumours, it is noted, which are often fatal, are very rare in women of childbearing age. The evidence for an association between the tumours and the pill, it is admitted, is by no means watertight. 'Nevertheless', *The Lancet* comments, 'an up-to-date assessment of the risk of hepatoma [liver tumour] in women on oral contraceptives would be welcome.'

Herbs that heal

Is it possible that in the variegated assortment that Nature has to offer us among the herbs of the world there may be some substance that will prevent procreation without any hazards to the woman taking it? It is certainly a search worth undertaking. Interference with the hormonal balance is not the only method of birth control, and the mere fact that it has caught the fancy of the pharmaceutical industry is no excuse for maintaining it without any attempt to discover other and safer methods of achieving the same aim. The world population problem is such an explosively emotive subject that the still small voice of medical caution has tended to be drowned amid the raucous amplifiers of the politicians, sociologists and other do-good hangers-on. It is time that the modern descendants of Hippocrates refused to behave in this sheep-like manner and turned to Nature to search for some alternative to the much-vaunted 'pill'.

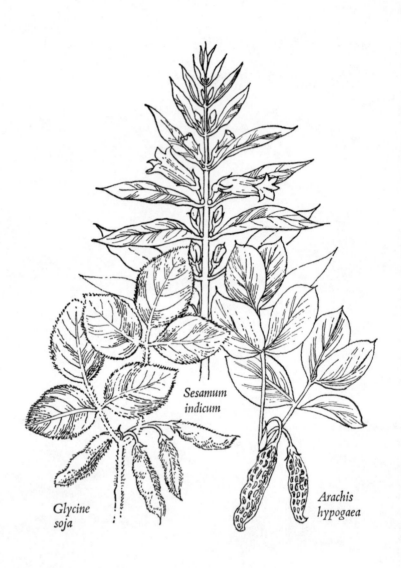

Sesamum
indicum

Glycine
soja

Arachis
hypogaea

11
Herbs that nourish

Prevention is better than cure: the latter-day medical adaptation of the old adage that 'a stitch in time saves nine', has been paid so much lip-service by doctors that it has been wellnigh licked into oblivion. This is scarcely surprising. Traditionally doctors are trained to cure, not to prevent, disease. All the sentiment of Sir Luke Fildes' bedside vigil, all the glamour of the operating theatre, all the drama of the patient snatched from the jaws of death: these are the highlights of traditional medicine and what have attracted so many to its ranks over the years. Preventive medicine, on the other hand, represents the chores of medicine: drains and sewer farms, knackers' yards and slaughter houses (abattoirs in modern parlance), lousy heads and scabious skins.

The post-1945 era, however, has seen a change in this traditional heirloom. As pollution, overbreeding and underfeeding have become the modern horsemen of the apocalypse, doctors have begun to realize that prevention must take priority over cure, and that, if the human race is to achieve any of those attributes of ful-filment that have stirred the soul of man since his creation, then a reorientation of the practice of medicine is called for. Such a reorientation will take time, but in principle it has been accepted.

It is therefore only logical that this final chapter should be devoted to the contribution of herbs and plants to the prevention of disease by providing a richer, fuller diet for the teeming millions struggling for existence on the face of the earth. Only some of the more recent and promising developments in this sphere will be dealt with but, in order to keep a link with the historical past and thereby preserve that sense of perspective which is so essential to a balanced review of the future, a brief reference may first be allowed to one of the oldest means of supplementing the diet of mankind: namely, manna. Strictly speaking this is a generic term applied to the saccharine exudations from a number of different plants belonging to various natural orders, but at the present day, unless otherwise specified, it is taken to mean the saccharine exudation from the stems of the manna ash, or flowering ash (*Fraxinus ornus*), a small tree widely distributed over southern Europe and cultivated in Sicily for the production of manna. When the trees are ten years old, transverse cuts are made in the trunk, from which comes a sugary exudate which is either removed on a stick or tiles, or allowed to dry when it is removed in flakes. Its main constituent is mannitol, a carbohydrate. It has a pleasant smell and a sweet taste, and its chief use nowadays is as a laxative for infants and children.

Other sources of manna include several species of *Tamarix*, which grows widely in the Near East, and in which the manna is exuded as a result of the tree being wounded by an insect. Manna may also be obtained from several other plants, including the European birch (*Larix decidua*) and some conifers.

Biblical manna, which is described in *Exodus* as being 'like coriander seed, white; and the taste of it like wafers made with honey', was probably the desert lichen, *Lecanora esculenta*, which can be carried for long distances by the wind, though other suggestions are that it may have been a fungus, or tamarix manna. Even today in the Middle East manna is still collected and eaten as a sweetmeat.

There may not seem to be much connection between the manna of the great exodus of circa 1500 BC and the feeding of the hungry millions of 1975 AD by protein rescued from the haulm of modern crops, but they are united in their common aim of finding the wherewithal to keep body and soul together. Today we may be somewhat more scientific in our approach to the problem of malnutrition and starvation. Certainly it is now appreciated that what is missing from the diets of a large proportion of the millions of Asia and Africa is protein. Carbohydrate is relatively easy to come by, and fat is not too tricky a problem. Neither of these, however, is sufficient for healthy growth unless supplemented by protein upon which we, and particularly the growing child, are dependent for certain amino-acids, as they are known, which are essential building bricks for muscle, bone and the like.

Flesh, in the form of meat, fish or game is the best source of protein, along with eggs and milk: but all these are expensive, with the exception of skimmed milk, of which the EEC is piling up mountains comparable with those it has of beef, butter and other essential (and in other parts of the world badly needed) foodstuffs. Next in order of priority as a source of protein come the pulses, such as peas, beans and lentils. All these, however, are not sufficient to meet world demand, and attention has therefore been turned to the protein in the leaves and stems of plants. These are obviously a rich source, it having been estimated that in some cases the protein content of the discarded haulm (that is, the stems, stalks and leaves) of crop plants may be as great as that of the harvested crop.

The knowledge that leaves contain protein is not new, and dates back a couple of hundred years, but it was only some fifty years ago that the suggestion was seriously put forward that this leaf protein might be used as food. An attempt to develop this in a big way was made in Britain, mainly at the Rothamsted Experimental Station at Harpenden in Hertfordshire, during the 1939–45 War, but with little practical success. Since then, however, the growing shortage of protein has given a fresh impetus and investigations are now being carried out in many parts of the world, particularly Britain, Sweden, India, New Zealand and the USA.

The approach has been a twofold one. One has been the growing of crops especially to see how much protein could be obtained from them: cereals and clover, for example, at Rothamsted, and lucerne in the USA and New Zealand. Up to three tons of protein per hectare (approximately two and a half acres) annually have been obtained in this way. In addition, protein has been obtained from twenty or thirty other species, many of them classed as weeds, and it has been forecast that before long many plants hitherto classed as weeds will be grown for their protein content. One of the more important and immediate targets, however, is all the plant material now being treated as waste. Thus, it has been estimated that around 60,000 tons of protein is being wasted annually in Britain alone by destroying haulm instead of harvesting it. The waste in this respect with sugar beet is the most scandalous of all. Yet another interesting comparison that has been made is that more protein can be extracted from the haulm of peas picked for canning and freezing than is present in the peas as they reach the public.

One of the practical difficulties is that of evolving a commercially viable method of extracting the protein but Dr N W Pirie, the British pioneer in this field, has recently described a method of extraction which is so simple that it could be a small-scale industry in any community able to manage a tractor. That this is all practical politics, and not merely academic theorizing, is indicated by the report of a six-month experiment, in which schoolchildren on a diet consisting basically of ragi (finger or African millet), which is cultivated as a food crop in China, India and Central Africa, were given supplements of ten grams of protein daily in the form of either lucerne leaf protein or sesame seed. On the basis of the weight, height and haemoglobin content of the blood, the children on leaf protein did better than those on sesame seed, even though the protein in the latter is regarded as one of the best sources of seed, or pulse, protein.

Unfortunately, much of this excellent protein in sesame seeds is also wasted, all the emphasis having been on the oil extracted from them. Known also as Gingelly oil or Teel oil, it has a slight pleasant odour and a bland taste, and properties comparable to those of olive oil. So much is it valued in Asia and Africa that it is now one of the most important sources of fat in these continents, being widely cultivated in China, India, Nigeria and the Sudan. The seeds contain some 50% oil and 15%–20% protein. The snag is that hitherto most of the protein has been left in the residue when the oil has been pressed from the seeds. This, however, has not been a complete loss as the residue is made into cattle cake.

On the other hand, this is not the most satisfying way of dealing with the matter in these days of protein shortage, especially as the residue contains 50% protein. The matter was therefore taken up at the National College of Technology in Weybridge. Their first observation was that the residue contained too much fibre and oxalic acid to make it fit for human consumption. Their second observation was that both these undesirable factors were present mainly in the outer coat of the seed. The problem therefore was to get rid of the fibre and oxalic acid, and this they did by evolving a way of treating the outer coat with an alkali solution so that it could be easily removed before the oil was extracted. This worked, and the residue, after the extraction of the oil, now contained only a small harmless proportion of fibre and oxalic acid. In this way yet another source of protein has been effectively tapped for human consumption.

The Weybridge researchers then went on to the problem of the waste from the processing of palm oil. This is now done on an increasingly large scale in Malaya and elsewhere, and disposal of the waste is their major pollution problem. It is apparently a nasty, thick, brown viscous waste which is discharged into rivers and streams where it is causing considerable trouble for the farmers who use the water for irrigation. The Weybridge workers have worked out a method of using this waste to grow fungi which have high nutritive value and could be used as food for pigs and poultry. This they have achieved on a small scale in the laboratory with two species of fungi, and hope to be able to develop the technique to a full commercial scale in two or three years. If they succeed with palm oil waste, then they propose to turn their attention to the comparable waste from olive oil in Greece and Italy and sisal waste in East Africa, all of which present a pollution problem, and in all of which there is wastage of precious protein·

Soya bean is another rich source of protein (twice as high as most other pulses) which hitherto has never been fully utilized outside China. Although it has been cultivated in China since around 3000 BC when there are written accounts of its cultivation, it was not introduced to Europe till the seventeenth century and to North America in the early years of the last century. Outside China no attempt was made to exploit it until the turn of the present century, but now nearly thirty million tons of the beans are produced annually: around 60% in China, 35% in the USA, and the remainder in central Europe, India and Indonesia.

As a source of protein it compares very favourably with beef. Thus, a steer eats 1200 pounds of crude protein a year to produce 75 pounds of meat protein, and to produce this amount it would have had to be fed the equivalent of two acres of soya bean.

Put another way, soya bean yields 570 pounds of protein per acre, compared with only 38 pounds in the form of meat. The technical problems to be overcome in converting soya-bean protein into an acceptable imitation of meat are considerable, but they are now being tackled successfully. One of the first ways of using it was in vegetable milk substitutes, which are now being tried to an increasing extent in India, Africa and South America. It is now being tested in school meals in Britain, incorporated as a meat substitute, and is also becoming generally available to the public.

Peanuts, or groundnuts (to give them the name which was used for the catastrophic experiment by the British Government to develop them as a major profit-making industry in Tanzania, which brought handsome rewards to the entrepreneurs and lashings of food to the local inhabitants), are another plant source of food which has never been fully exploited. Hitherto they have been used mainly for the oil content which is high, the whole seeds, or nuts, containing 40% fat – twice as much as soya bean. This is used mainly as a cooking oil and for making margarine and soap. The residue, once the oil has been expressed, is used only as cattle cake in spite of the fact that it is an excellent source of protein. This seems to be mainly because of its unpleasant taste, which is literally nauseating.

The food technologists, however, are now on to the problem and have already succeeded in incorporating up to 10% of the residue in flour from millets, wheat and other sources, as well as making other palatable foods in which an appreciable amount of the protein has come from groundnut protein.

It owes its name of groundnut to the fact that after flowering the ends of the stalks bend down and the young pods are forced into the soil where they ripen underground and have to be harvested by digging. The plant, which is indigenous to Brazil, was cultivated extensively by the Incas and Mayas, and brought by the Spaniards to Europe and Africa, whence it spread to the East. Today groundnuts are cultivated in Africa, India, China and America, and constitute the third largest source in the world of fixed oil. In the USA they were ignored until the hard-pushed and semi-starved Union soldiers during the Civil War discovered they were a useful source of food and roasted them over their camp fires. They retained their taste for them in civilian life and gradually, especially under the encouragement of George Washington Carver, the distinguished botanist and statesman, they became a major crop of the Southern States. Today no foodstore in the USA is complete without peanuts in some form or other, whether it be peanut butter, peanut meal or merely roasted peanuts.

While peanuts, or groundnuts, have been looming ever larger on the nutritional front, the oil they produce, arachis oil, has been attracting attention in an entirely different field. It was some twenty years ago that it was first noticed that the arachis oil base in which an experimental anti-inflammatory drug was being administered to animals had itself an anti-inflammatory action. The next observation was that the injection of arachis oil lengthened the incubation period of experimental scrapie (a troublesome nervous disease of unknown origin in sheep) in mice. The sequel to this was the demonstration that arachis oil and some other plant oils contained potent anti-inflammatory components quite apart from fatty acids.

The exciting possibility now is that this may have some application to two of the most distressing diseases in our midst, of neither of which we know the cause: namely, multiple sclerosis and Parkinsonism. Both these conditions come into the category of what are known as slow encephalopathies, which include the experimental and animal diseases in which arachis and other plant oils have given the results just recounted. In the words of a recent and authoritative review of the subject in *The Lancet*:

'Some plant oils and other lecithin-rich foods, such as egg-yolk, seem to contain pharmacologically active trace substances with anti-inflammatory effects comparable to, and more powerful than, that of cortisone.'

All this is rather vague and it is much too early to build up any hopes but, when dealing with two such incurable, crippling and relatively common diseases, it would be equally wrong to ignore the possibilities altogether. There is certainly no immediate application of this work, either dietetic or medicinal. On the other hand, it does mean that yet another gleam of hope has been raised which may lead on to further advances in the elucidation of these two mysterious diseases.

To grow plants efficiently it is necessary to protect them against predators. Nature in the raw is the ever-present inverse of the smiling benign Nature, with its lovely flowers, its verdant meadows and its golden corn, that we like to picture. Man is not the only member of Nature interested in food crops: insects and other predators, as we disdainfully name them, are just as interested, and, unless we protect crops against them there will be little left for humanity to exist on. They may not all be as sweeping in their onslaughts as the locust, but they can cause enough damage to make the difference between existence and starvation.

Fortunately, Nature herself supplies a most efficient insecticide in the form of *Chrysanthemum cinerariaefolium*, better known as pyrethrum flower or insect flower. From this is obtained pyrethrum, one of the most efficient insecticides, or pesticides, we possess. As so often happens as to be almost monotonous in the telling, the use of pyrethrum powder against insects was known to the ancient Chinese. It was also known in Persia, where the plant is called the insect flower, and for a long time the Persians kept this information to themselves as a carefully guarded secret. During the last century Yugoslavia, or Dalmatia as it was then known, where the plant is indigenous, became the chief source of supply and, as the demand increased, its cultivation spread to other parts of Europe, America and Japan.

Today, however, Kenya is the main source of origin, supplying over 70% of the world demand. This is a most impressive record in view of the fact that it was only in the later 1920s that a British settler imported seed from Dalmatia and started growing it. From the beginning it was a success, the flowers blooming almost all the year round in the cool sunny highlands. The first cash crop was harvested in 1933 and, by 1935, 327 tons were being produced. Today the figure has grown to 16,000 tons, valued at £8 million. The rest of the world supply comes principally from Tanzania, Rwanda, Ecuador and New Guinea.

In recent years pyrethrum has had a somewhat variegated career on account of the competing claims of DDT and the other synthetic insecticides or pesticides that swept the world after the 1939–45 War. The Kenyans, however, refused to give up growing this lucrative crop. The price might fall, but they were going to carry on. How right they were. Those much vaunted man-made insecticides were soon put in their place by Nature which started producing insects and pests resistant to them; and recently the demand for pyrethrum has started rising again, growing from an annual average of 14,300 tons in 1962–66 to around 21,000 tons in 1975.

Its claims to fame are manifold. It is rapidly toxic to a wide range of insects, including mosquitoes, greenflies and houseflies, as well as grain weevils and flour beetles, not to mention moths. It has an almost instantaneous knock-out effect by virtue of its action on the nervous system, resulting in convulsions and paralysis. In this respect it has a much quicker killing action than DDT and such insecticides, but it is less persistent and less stable. For this reason it is sometimes combined in aerosols with DDT or gamma benzene hexachloride (lidane), such mixtures giving a quick knock-down action with a more lasting effect. Just as important as all this is the fact that it is harmless to warm-blooded animals.

Today therefore this invaluable herb ('pretty little flowers with yellow centres', as they have been described) which heals by helping to provide mankind with an adequate supply of food, as well as protecting him from the ravages of disease-bearing insects such as mosquitoes, is coming back into its own. It is being used increasingly widely in domestic and agricultural insecticidal sprays and dusting powers, in the form of mosquito coils, and as a non-inflammable spray for use in aircraft to kill insect vectors and so prevent the transmission of insect-borne diseases.

So we complete this herbal circle of healing, prevention and nutrition: a three-in-one circle which we so often ignore – and to our cost. Circumnavigating it has been a most revealing process, demonstrating once again how we ignore Nature at a price. The fact that, according to Holy Script, we are made in the image of God, is no excuse for ignoring Nature. We are part and parcel of her, and it is by co-operating with her and exploring her mysteries that we are most likely to live the life we all desire, and to have it more abundantly.

This is no mere idle philosophical fancy, with the slogan of 'back to Nature'. It is an integration of mind, body and spirit which is much more likely to fulfil our hopes and ambitions than the arid atmosphere in which the modern synthesist, whether chemist, pharmacologist or biologist, spends his life, resembling in so many ways the alchemist of old in his arid futile search for gold. The psalmist's 'riches of the earth' are ours. Why then do we not explore them for what they are producing in the way of herbs that heal?

Bibliography

Ackerknecht, Erwin H. *Therapeutics. From the Primitives to the 20th Century*, 1973

Bowles, E. A. *A Handbook of Crocus and Colchicum for Gardeners*, 1952

Camp, John *Magic, Myth and Medicine*, 1974

Clair, Colin *Of Herbs and Spices*, 1961

Culpeper, Nicholas *The Complete Herbal*, 1653

Flückiger, Friedrich A. and Hanbury, Daniel *Pharmacographia. A History of the Principal Drugs of Vegetable Origin Met With in Great Britain and British India*, 2nd edition, 1879

Grigson, Geoffrey *The Englishman's Flora*, 1955

Hemphill, Rosemary *Herbs for All Seasons*, 1975

Howes, F. N. *A Dictionary of Useful and Everyday Plants and Their Common Names*, 1974

Keys, Thomas E. *The History of Surgical Anesthesia*, 1963

Kreig, Margaret B. *Green Medicine*, 1965

Lehner, E. & J. *Folklore and Odysseys of Food and Medicinal Plants*, 1973

Li, C. P. *Chinese Herbal Medicine*, 1974

Loewenfeld, Claire and Back, Phillips *The Complete Book of Herbs and Spices*, 1974

Major, Ralph H. *A History of Medicine*, 1954

Mességué, Maurice *Of Men and Plants*, 1972

Mez-Mangold, Lydia *A History of Drugs*, 1971

Mortimer, Phyllis *Only When It Hurts. Being a Curious Collection of Old Fashioned Remedies and Dissertations on Matters of Health*, 1974

Peck, T. Whitemore and Wilkinson, Douglas *William Withering of Birmingham*, 1950

Porter, Enid *The Folklore of East Anglia*, 1974

Quinn, Joseph R. (Ed.) *Medicine and Public Health in the People's Republic of China*, 1973

Quinn, Joseph R. (Ed.) *China Medicine As We Saw It*, 1974

Rubin, Stanley *Medieval English Medicine*, 1974

Sanecki, Kay N. *The Complete Book of Herbs*, 1974

Singer, Charles and Underwood, E. Asher *A Short History of Medicine*, 2nd edition, 1962

Step, Edward *Herbs and Healing*, 1926

Swain, Tony (Ed.) *Plants in the Development of Modern Medicine*, 1972

Usher, George *A Dictionary of Plants Used by Man*, 1974

Index

Index

Index